Gum Disease:
The Silent Battle
in Your Mouth

Natural Ways To Keep Your Mouth Healthy
And Minimise Future Dental Appointments

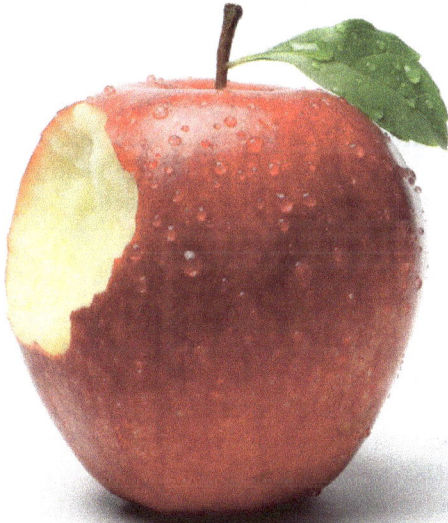

Dr. Elmar Jung & Graeme Dinnen

What Your Dentist Should Be Telling You:
A Few Words First....

You're about to discover a variety of ways to help keep your teeth and gums in a condition you didn't think possible. As a result, this will be one of the most crucial documents you'll ever read on the subject. Print and bind a copy to keep for future use, freely passing it on to friends and family if you think they'll benefit from it, even in some small way. They'll love you for it.

It's all too easy to overlook that our bodies are holistic, interconnected marvels that thrive only when each part hums in harmony. What you introduce into your mouth profoundly impacts your entire being. A pristine mouth isn't merely a visual delight; it's vital for lifelong health.

Regarding excitement, reading about teeth and gums is up there alongside listening to 16th-century Spanish Organ music (with abject apologies to any 16th-century organ grinders). So, I'll keep the technical bits to a minimum, although some things have to be explained.

I can educate you, but I can't do it for you. That's your job, but it'll be much easier now. I've put together a boot camp approach to dental health. Read and try out the information in a manner that's seriously close to enthusiasm, and you'll have mastered the basics. Your dentist is unlikely to have told you much of what we write about. Not their fault - it just isn't part of their training. It would still be prudent to visit your dentist and hygienist, but you're not likely to need as much remedial action as often as before.

It's not my place to answer questions on what type of dental work you should have. That I leave to your dentist, but if you don't pay attention here, you'll soon be lying back in that reclining chair hearing the words "*Open Wide!*"

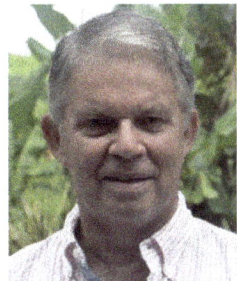

Graeme Dinnen

Co-Author Dr. Elmar Jung, DDS

In my 30 years as a holistic dentist I have witnessed life-saving dental work as well as dental work that was totally unnecessary.

I highly recommend "Gum Disease: The Silent Battle In Your Mouth" because when your mouth is under attack, you can be confident that being armed with the right knowledge will help you take responsibility in introducing the necessary measures to combat gum disease.

Even arming yourself in a preventative capacity, you can be assured that this one little book can lead to a healthy mouth and healthy you. Understand the cause of your condition, and it becomes easier for you to do something about it.

Ensure that during your dental appointments the dentist discusses what may have triggered your condition and what you can do to ensure it doesn't recur.

By reading "Gum Disease: The Silent Battle In Your Moutb" you'll be tapping into a valuable source of information for you and your family. The recommendations given will help you understand the crucial importance of your dental health and what can (and usually will) go wrong if deterioration of any nature sets in.

You will also gain enormous benefit from the encouragement to eat and drink sensibly, using botanicals and other non-drug approaches as a preventative measure to sustain dental and ultimately overall health.

The information is here. The rest is up to you.

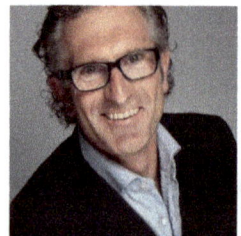

Dr Elmar Jung
Author: 'Shut Your Mouth And Open Wide'

Preliminaries

If I give you many different natural mouthwashes to choose from, or a similar number of toothpastes to make at home, you may only ever make a few of them. Once you've mastered two or three, there's no need to learn any more, although your natural instinct to experiment may prove me wrong.

I won't list the scientific properties of every botanical or remedy I recommend because the more there is to read, the less likely people are to do so. If you need specifics on something, use your browser.

I will provide you with a wide range of natural approaches to keep your mouth healthy. After that, it's up to your wanton experimentation.

You may think, "What would the toothpaste taste like if I added some peppermint oil?"; "Would it be more effective if I added unrefined sea salt to increase the mineral content and make the concoction slightly more abrasive?" or "Would olive oil be better than coconut oil as a base for toothpaste?"

Questionable research carried out in 2016 claimed that humans have an 8-second attention span on the internet. In 2000, it used to be 12 seconds. As the same research showed, goldfish have a 9-second attention span, and we humans have a shorter attention span than goldfish. Given the reputation of goldfish, if true, that's alarming. I didn't know goldfish used the internet!

It's time to silence the background music and turn off all social media. Read this actively. Try out the recommendations, and the health of your mouth will transform. That's the only assurance I can give you.

Congratulations on getting this far. You've sailed past the 8-second test!

Like most people, you probably dread the prospect of even minor gum surgery. For years, you've unquestioningly followed the advice of your dentist to brush more, floss more and rinse with mouthwash, yet at your next appointment, your dentist finds yet another small cavity or locates gum deterioration and insists it must be dealt with before things get worse.

Despite this you're still told that you need to brush more, floss more and rinse with mouthwash more. Is this designed to keep us as repeat, paying customers?

Old Dental sayings:

- You don't have to clean all your teeth - only the ones you want to keep.
- The toothbrush doesn't remove six months of tartar 30 minutes before your dental appointment!
- Dentistry is not expensive, neglect is.

Contents

Faith, Hope & Clarity

The purpose of this ebook is to give you renewed hope for a problem-free mouth. You don't have to experiment with every recipe or recommendation, but don't be afraid to try any of them. Just because you've never heard of activated charcoal or been told that turmeric will probably stain your kitchen, they're poor reasons not to try them. I've used them often (and been told to clean up afterwards). They're all simple to use.

One issue with ebooks is that only a few people read them right through. I, too, have been guilty of that. Had I written an exhaustive document extolling the virtues of every botanical remedy, I wouldn't have done readers a favour. Already, there is more than sufficient information to build and maintain a vastly improved sense of dental health, so much so that when you use these suggestions, you'll not only have the opportunity to have much healthier teeth and gums but there's a likelihood you'll only need to visit the dentist or hygienist for emergencies or occasional cleanings and inspections.

I invite you to take full responsibility for caring for your teeth. The alternative is not worth considering.

Can Brushing & Flossing CAUSE Gum Disease?

In the words of Dr Joseph Phillips, DDS (1922 - 2003)

"There's not much information out there that gives people a choice on how to care for their mouths. There's brushing and flossing and a million different kinds of brushes and toothpastes and flosses with which to do this, which brings us back to basic brushing and flossing. Bearing in mind that 90% of all adults in the Western world suffer from some degree of gum disease (yes, children too), and most people over 60 have no teeth at all, is brushing and flossing the answer?

Of course, no matter how well you clean your teeth, your mouth still remains 90% dirty, as teeth occupy only 10% of the surface of your mouth. So it is just as essential to clean the gums, cheeks, roof, floor, and tongue. Learn how to eliminate bad breath without mouthwash.

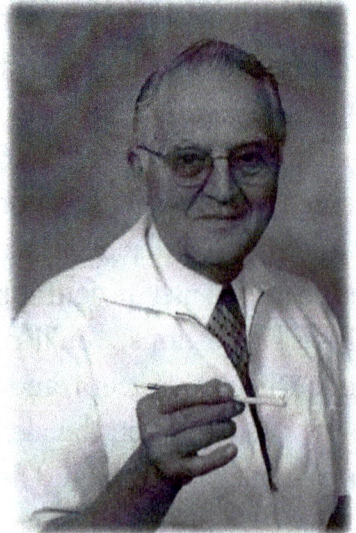

"My sincere belief is that a dentist can keep your teeth for you only by teaching you to help yourself."

-Dr. J.E. Phillips

If your dentist says, "You have to brush more because you have a plaque on your teeth." The next time you see him, he says, "You have to brush still more and floss more because your gums are bleeding," and he suggests that you see the hygienist more often for cleaning your teeth, you will soon be a candidate for deep curettage and periodontal (gum) surgery.

Frequent brushing and flossing, cleaning by the hygienist, and gum surgery never cure periodontal disease. As time passes, this leads to more curettage, surgery, and eventually, tooth extraction.

Brushing and flossing can cause periodontal disease. Cleaning under the gums daily will prevent the disease from starting and, in most cases, heal the gums.

It would be best if you did not brush your teeth unless you can clean the sulcus out afterwards. By the way, brushing is only for cosmetics. As dentistry has insisted that people brush more, periodontal disease has attacked much younger people with gingivitis (bleeding gums). This is the precursor to periodontal disease.

The Freddy Krueger
Of Your Mouth

Your alarm has just gone off. This is your wake-up call. From this moment on, it's time to strap yourself in and pay attention because what you read here is critical to your health. I'm not talking about the health of just your mouth; this is vital information for the well-being of your entire body.

Remember that up to 80% of diseases are believed to originate in the mouth, so stay with me here.

Whether you know this or not, one word holds more terror than the thought of Dracula, Frankenstein and Freddy Krueger combined.

That word is PERIODONTITIS (per-e-o-don-TIE-tis). If you've heard the phrase before but weren't 100% sure what it means, you're about to find out. You will only appreciate why I'm telling you about this right at the start.

The stages of periodontal disease

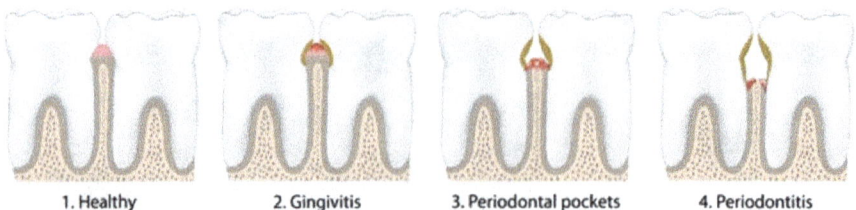

1. Healthy   2. Gingivitis   3. Periodontal pockets   4. Periodontitis

4

Look up a dictionary definition of periodontitis, and you'll read that it's a severe gum infection that can destroy the bone and damage the soft tissue supporting your teeth. In the long term, it can cause your teeth to fall out.

These definitions don't convey the horror of what can happen to the rest of your body when periodontitis sets in. And yes, periodontitis and tooth loss are closely linked with oral cancers. (Michaud DS, Liu Y, Meyer M, Giovannucci E, Joshipura K. Periodontal disease, tooth loss, and cancer risk in male health professionals: a prospective cohort study. Lancet Oncol 2008; 9: 550-558).

The good news is that periodontitis is preventable. Hang on a moment. If it's preventable, why is it so common? The dictionary definitions say it's predominantly the result of poor oral hygiene.

Let me explain plainly: You're not cleaning your teeth and gums properly!

Next time you clean your teeth, note how long you brush for. If under 3 minutes, you may be a candidate for periodontitis. And just maybe that's why the statistics show that 47% of people in the USA have mild, moderate, or severe periodontitis, this percentage rising to 70% in those over 65 years old. That statistic is beyond serious.

As well as suffering from periodontitis, approximately one-third of adults in the world now suffer needlessly from tooth decay.

Microorganisms are opportunistic invaders taking advantage of what's on offer, but are NOT the real cause of the problem.

Many dentists will claim that brushing and flossing at least twice a day and getting regular dental checkups will reduce your chances of developing periodontitis and tooth decay and, should it develop, significantly improve the probability of treating it successfully.

And these dentists are right....but there's more.

Brushing and flossing daily and rinsing with mouthwash isn't all that's needed. For example, if you don't brush properly, you may just be pushing plaque from one part of your mouth to another. The way in which you've been cleaning your teeth all your life may be doing more damage than you know.

Read on to find out what you can do instead that's so much better than the traditional brushing, toothpaste, flossing, and mouthwashing methods you've been using so far.

I suggest this because periodontitis results from microorganisms sticking to and growing on the surface of your teeth. To establish the level of bone loss and locate the presence and extent of periodontitis, dentists probe the soft gum tissue around the base of the teeth.

Removing these sticky microorganisms must be done daily and properly; traditional brushing with toothpaste doesn't do everything that's necessary. Put another way, if brushing and flossing were as effective as is claimed, people wouldn't develop periodontitis.

I'll leave you with that thought. Right now, we need to get you on the right track. I will first build a background wall of information so that all the subsequent pieces can fit into place and remain there.

There's a video that really addresses the periodontitis issue, both in terms of understanding and what you can do about it. If you genuinely want to find the motivation to keep your mouth healthy, put aside the hour; your eyes will be opened and your jaw will drop.

I'm writing this in BOLD because YOU NEED TO WATCH IT

I can think of nothing better than watching this clip made available by the Functional Oral Summit.

Key in to your browser and watch '**Functional Oral Health Summit: Say Ahh!**' OK it's 59:54 minutes long yet is highly motivating.

The *'Say Aah!'* title doesn't make you want to jump for joy, but the information explains the damage caused by gum disease if left to decay. Most people (not you, of course!) do nothing about it until it's almost too late, which is why gum disease is the most common poor health condition humans suffer.

Here's an excerpt: Jeanne Dockins, Operating Room Nurse, is passionate about her patients' safety.

> *"One lady told me...I asked her if she had periodontal disease and she said "Yes" she knew she had it but that it was expensive to treat (and) she didn't have dental insurance. She was having a total knee (replacement) put in.*
>
> *So she had her total knee, she went home. A few months later she got infected (and) they had to take her knee out. Then she had to live without a knee for a while.*
>
> *Then they had to put a new knee back in; it got infected. They took it out and when I was her nurse, two years later they were amputating her*

leg. And she didn't know anything about periodontal disease but she had an infection and when she went into surgery her husband told me that the cost of their medical bill for the past 2 years was two million dollars"

You'll also listen to Dr David Verity giving you reasons why you should never have surgery while you have periodontal disease. In the USA, up to 50% of people who go into hospital for surgery already suffer from periodontal disease.

Watch the film. If you don't have time today, make time tomorrow. Don't skip this. It'll change your approach to dental health completely.

There's also information on how periodontitis can affect sleep apnea and cancer.

Remember while you're watching this - your mouth is the dirtiest part of your body, causing morbidity and mortality, usually through chronic inflammation (i.e. gum disease).

Part One:

The Value Of
A Healthy Mouth

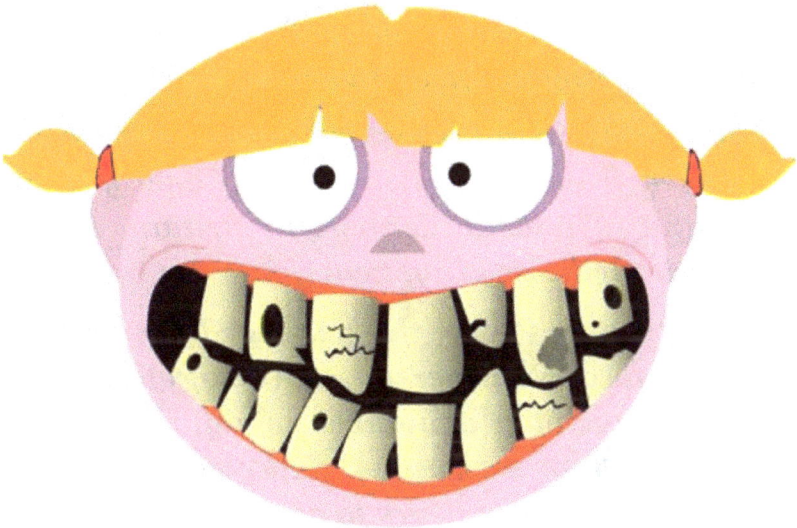

There are billions of bacteria in your mouth - more than the number of humans on earth. And like humans, some are friendly; others are not so friendly. The condition of your mouth is a window into the health of your body. Indeed, most chronic or infectious diseases that trouble us today are influenced by the health of our mouths.

If you have poor dental health, you will have other health problems. Any experienced dentist can ask you to say "Ahhhh" and quickly see what condition the rest of your body is in.

A man goes to the dentist and says, "I've got a terrible toothache". The dentist takes one look at the tooth and says, "There's nothing wrong with that tooth. You need to get your intestines cleaned out". The man undergoes colonic irrigation and the pain in the tooth disappears.

Another man who's pulled a hamstring muscle goes to see his dentist for a check-up. The dentist makes a quick realignment of one of his teeth, and his hamstring problem is cured.

These seemingly fantastical cases are just a few selected from the patient files of one of a small handful of holistic dentists in Britain. In itself, holistic medicine is not new.

In the 1980s, it was the buzzword for seeing the patient as a whole person, and also referred to the integration of a a number of different medical systems, both alternative and conventional. The concept has taken years to arrive in the relatively staid world of the dental profession."

from What Doctors Don't Tell You

Inside your mouth are teeth, gums, tongue, cheeks, tonsils, glands, bones, muscles, that dangly uvula, and about 700 species of bacteria, all fighting for survival. The odd fungus will lurk together with a cache of parasites and a virus or two. What keeps you healthy is when the parasites are mostly eliminated and everything else is in balance. This is the state of homeostasis.

Consider What You're Eating

This is not a guide to better eating habits. Plenty of differing opinions on this subject are already available in books and magazines, many of which rate their opinions over the facts. Looking after yourself is a long-term project, so you must fill yourself with the right ingredients to have any real chance of watching your grandchildren grow up.

The simplest analogy is this: If you put cheap motor oil in a Ferrari, you won't get the engine performance you want. The same goes for food; fill yourself with burgers, pizzas, and sodas, and your body may not function as you want it to.

Everything in life is about balance - Yin and Yang, night and day, female and male, hot and cold. Today would be a good time to begin balancing any nutritional debt you may have built up......because it's slowly harming you.

If I sound like I'm nagging, I probably am. Try chewing your food a little more than you probably do now. If your food is improperly masticated, it can't provide the nutrients required for the cellular support and regeneration your body craves.

Today's foods are so compromised in terms of being mushed and overcooked before they are eaten that there is little left to do for your teeth.

Like any other body part, teeth must be exercised to be appropriately preserved. To feel invigorated and to keep blood circulation active, teeth also need stimulating pressure from crunchy fruit (apples), vegetables (carrots), and even toothbrush tree sticks (I'll cover these later).

Killer whales in captivity have broken teeth because they're not chasing and killing their prey as Nature intended. Their meals are tossed into the air for them to gulp down in exchange for crowd-pleasing acrobatics.

There is a purpose to chewing. It releases enzymes that help break down the food you're eating. Some enzymes come from the food; the rest are produced in your saliva.

If you aren't chewing sufficiently to draw the enzymes out of the food, think of it as borrowing tomorrow's enzymes to digest today's food. This may be news to you, but:

- the quality of food you eat can impact the health of your mouth.
- the quality of food you eat can impact the health of your mouth MORE THAN brushing your teeth does,
- If you eat the right food, brushing should become a cosmetic exercise.

It is difficult these days to recommend a food without someone explaining why it may affect your metabolism and weight gain. Here I'm suggesting a selection of foods and beverages that can benefit your dental health.

If you have a specific condition, ask a nutritionist or your doctor whether this is appropriate for you. In terms of choice, everyone differs in what foods they like or dislike, so consider these recommendations as a guide.

Below are some helpful foods that are either rich in calcium, vitamins, phosphorous, antioxidants, probiotics, or just plain crunchy for your teeth. The list is not exhaustive, but it's worth migrating your food choices toward this list.

Beneficial Foods (preferably organic and not laced with GMOs)

- yogurt
- hard cheeses
- egg yolks
- wild-caught salmon
- fatty fishes
- red meats
- home-made bone broths (with gelatine)
- ginger soup
- almonds
- brazil nuts
- cashews
- black walnut
- pine nuts
- wholegrain
- nutmeg & mace
- pumpkin seeds
- sesame seeds
- chia seeds
- flax seeds
- leafy greens: broccoli
- kale
- spinach
- bamboo shoots
- bell peppers
- shiitake mushrooms
- beans
- tomatoes
- spinach
- apples
- berries
- carrots
- celery
- cucumbers
- figs
- kiwi fruit
- pears
- oranges
- grapes
- raisins
- rhubarb
- mangoes
- celery
- beetroot
- garlic
- ginger
- raw onions
- sweet potatoes
- avocado

- sauerkraut, miso, kimchi fermented vegetables/foods)
- wasabi (Japanese horse radish)
- mineral-rich unrefined sea salt

Big Brother in Your Shopping Basket

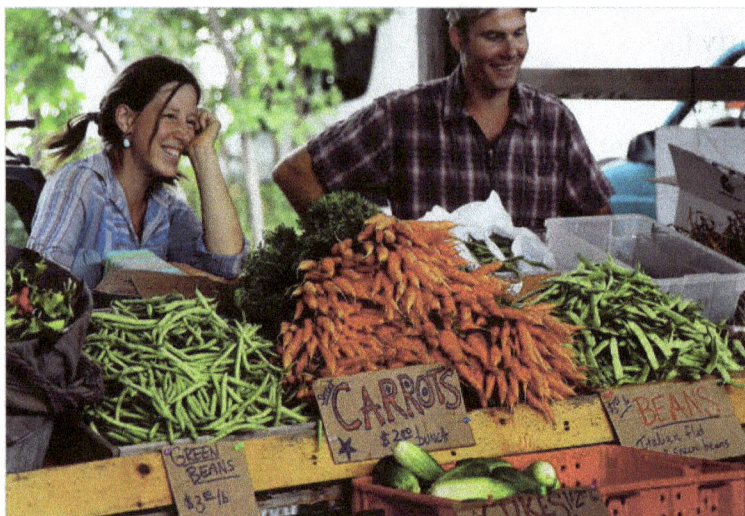

Wherever I can, I buy food from Farmer's Markets, where I've shaken hands with the people who grew it. So what if the carrot isn't straight? More important is that it hasn't been sprayed with questionable chemicals.

By shopping locally, I'm supporting human beings, not massive agribusiness conglomerates that grow heavily sprayed foods and devour details of my shopping habits through credit and loyalty cards to create demographic profiles that lure me back me with special offers I don't need.

Remember that the farmer rose early in the morning and toiled to grow that food. Buying from local farmers cuts out the middleman, allowing the farmer a regular cash flow. This sustains his family and allows them to re-invest in the business. When farmers sell to supermarkets, they are often paid months later, often at a meagre profit.

If you're looking for healthy food recommendations, the Weston A. Price Foundation has valuable information. Dr. Weston Price himself contributed so much to our current knowledge and understanding of dental health.

Random Food Tips:

- Spicy foods help stimulate salivary glands, ensuring you have sufficient saliva for eating.
- High-fibre foods can help increase the production of saliva in your mouth. As long as your mouth is healthy, saliva serves as a natural protector for teeth.
- Onions are rich in sulphur compounds that keep Streptococcus Mutans in check. They're powerful when eaten raw.
- Raw garlic helps to protect against tooth decay by inhibiting the fermentation of sugar (not recommended before a first date!).
- Eating Swiss or Cheddar cheese before a meal helps negate the acids that create plaque and stimulates saliva production. Eat more nuts! Chewing on cashew nuts will help eliminate rogue bacteria.
- Cashews are a heart-healthy source of zinc, magnesium, copper, phosphorus and manganese.
- Sugar, in most forms, is known to be a major contributor to cancer, but it doesn't stick to your teeth. Carbohydrates/

Starches do stick. While sugar has always had a bad press, bread, cereals, buns, pretzels, pasta, crackers, chips, muffins, cookies, and cakes are more significant contributors to dental decay and gum disease, especially if you're over 50 (like me). Consuming sugar upsets your body's calcium-to-phosphorous ratio. This leaches calcium and other essential minerals from your teeth and bones, thereby weakening them.

- Let's not forget the "apple-a-day" mantra you've heard since childhood. There's good reason for it (nutritional value and its valuable crunchiness for your teeth). Make sure it's organic.

According to author and medical medium Anthony William, eggs are great but become one of the foods you should be wary of if you're not feeling well. 'Suspect' eggs can feed the Epstein Barr Virus, but only if it is already present within you.

Pause here for thought. Who are you kissing goodnight? Are BOTH your mouths healthy? I'll cover this aspect later.

<u>Beneficial Drinks</u>

Red wine is on the beneficial list (yay!), but swallow it down. Allowing the wine to linger in your mouth isn't good for tooth enamel. Also helpful are black and green teas as they are believed to inhibit the formation of cavities and counteract the build-up of Streptococcus Mutants, a major contributor to those bacterial imbalances in your mouth.

Drink teas without adding sugar. If you find that difficult, try reducing the amount of sugar over a period.

Also beneficial are Oolong tea (valuable in the fight against parasites) and Kombucha, a lightly sweetened tea that the ancient Chinese considered the "Immortal Health Elixir" and has been around for more than 2,000 years.

Although some nutritionists claim coffee to be harmful and others extol its virtues, I suggest that if and when you drink coffee, you buy coffee beans and wash, dry, and grind them yourself. More than one high-street coffee chain has been caught serving customers with rancid beans. You deserve 'fresh', so make sure it is.

Raw cacao is always on my must-have list as it contains oxalic acid which helps prevent tooth decay. Remember to drink reasonable quantities of water daily to keep your saliva levels up.

Treat most fruit juices with suspicion, as the major brands tested have been found to contain glyphosate. Many red wines in California are being sprayed with glyphosate - sorry guys, I've enjoyed touring around your vineyards in Sonoma County, but if it's glyphosate you're spraying on the grapes, I'm voting against this practice with my wallet.

To avoid enamel damage from sugary drinks, use a straw if you absolutely have to drink them.

Once held sacred by ancient peoples, fermented Cod Liver Oil, a nutrient-dense source of Vitamins A and D and containing anti-inflammatory omega-3 fatty acids, helps build strong teeth and bones.

As the calcium in your teeth and bones is in constant flux, the Vitamin D helps to regulate the entire process. Cod liver oil and butter oil are a great way to remedy cavities, so when your dentist tells you there's a cavity forming and you need a filling, you know what to try next.

When calcium levels are low, calcium is no longer absorbed into teeth. To compensate for any calcium deficiency, the body leeches calcium from teeth. This alone could result in the early stages of periodontitis!

Calcium leeched out of the jaw results in bone loss but this does not necessarily cause periodontitis.

Key 'Dangers of Soy' into your browser for more information. I mentioned cheese earlier, but I hesitate before recommending any retail form of animal milk as it may be full of steroids and other questionable additives. Animal milk is designed for the animal's offspring, just as human mother's milk is intended for human babies.

My preference is not to drink or eat soy products unless they've been fermented.

Where I go shopping, there are alternatives such as almond, cashew, and coconut milk, but a cursory look at the labels for store-bought almond milk reveals only trace amounts of almonds. Why do they bother?

The school milk initiative needs to be revised. What's given to the kids contains the neurotoxin fluoride (even the Lancet and the Nationsl Institute of Health have questioned the toxicity of fluoride). Industrial fluoride should not be given to anyone, let alone schoolchildren.

One of my early morning drinks is a healthy pinch of unrefined, Celtic sea salt in a mug of hot water. I've been doing this for years, and it's unquestionably my preferred way of absorbing minerals and trace elements.

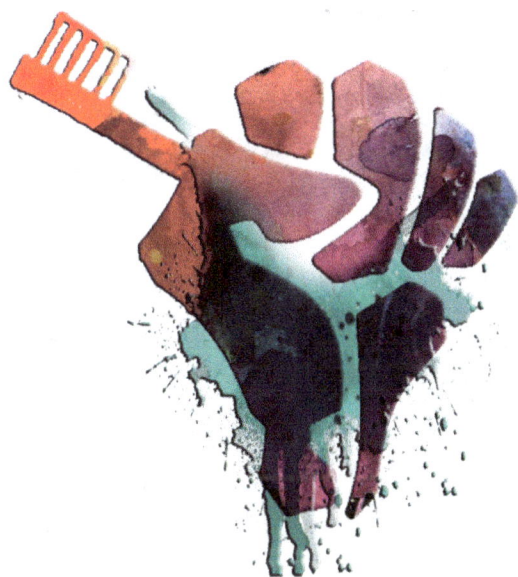

Part Two:

Your Teeth Are Alive

Despite what you may have been told, your teeth are ALIVE and in constant remineralisation, so let's keep them that way!

Please read that again, so it sinks in. Your teeth are A-L-I-V-E.

Saliva provides essential minerals to strengthen the tiny cells in your teeth. Your teeth are designed to last much longer than you are, so let's do what we can to ensure this happens. Caring for your teeth means so much more than just getting them white. It even helps prevent heart disease.

Archaeological digs have found several thousand-year-old skeletons, mostly with healthy teeth still intact. Indeed, part of the guess-how-old-this-skeleton-is process involves first examining the condition of the teeth. As an index of civilisation, the healthier the teeth are, the older the skeleton is likely to be.

> *"You can analyse a 30,000-year-old tooth and see something called the natal line. That shows when the baby came into the world and when it stopped feeding off of the placenta. And then we can tell when they are starting to wean and weaned just by looking at teeth and bones."*
> Hugh Milne, The Heart of Listening

You don't need to be like my Great Aunt Minnie (now on a cosmic holiday). When I stayed with her as a teenager, I'd come downstairs for breakfast and find her dentures staring at me from a glass of Steradent. That indelible vision alone encouraged me to look after my teeth better.

Suppose enamel is the toughest material that living organisms can produce and is so resistant. In that case, we have to seriously ask ourselves, why is it that in such a technologically advanced era, our teeth and gums are in such appalling condition?

There are several reasons. Let's start with a cross-section of how the teeth are made up (dull but necessary).

DENTINE
Dentine protects the pulp. It is the first layer under the enamel on the crown and the cementum on the root. It has a crystalline structure with millions of sponge-like openings or holes called 'Dentinal Tubules'.

PULP
Pulp is much like bone marrow - living connective tissue containing cells, nerves, blood and lymph vessels. If an infection in the pulp occurs, the pain can intensify, and the tooth could, at worst, die.

CEMENTUM
The surface of the root is called the cementum, a very thin layer that covers the dentine of the roots. There is no blood supply here.

ROOTS
The roots of your teeth are attached to your jawbone. This secures your teeth in place. Your front teeth and your canine

teeth normally have one root. Your premolars may have one or two roots. This is the most likely location for an abscess to develop. A neglected abscess can become a serious problem.

PERIODONTAL LIGAMENT

The tooth is not totally fixed in the bone but elastically joined to it by the periodontal ligament. This group of specialised connective tissue fibres essentially attach a tooth to the alveolar bone within which it sits. These ligaments also function as a buffer when you chew or grind your teeth.

Upper or Lower Teeth?

The downward force would normally determine that lower teeth contain more food and debris than upper teeth. Studies have shown that the upper teeth are far more susceptible to decay than the lower set as more protective saliva accumulates around the lower teeth. People spend less time brushing their upper teeth than their lower ones.

Cavities

For decades, we've read or been told that bacteria is the cause of cavities.

BACTERIA IS NOT THE ONLY CAUSE OF TOOTH CAVITIES

Many websites have yet to accept this material fact, putting them, as one writer suggested, *'in the modern age of dental barbarism."*

What Are The Real Causes Of Tooth Decay?

There are two schools of thought here. The first is that tooth decay is caused by poor-quality foods, and the second is that tooth decay is a childhood infection. Both approaches are well-researched and well-reasoned; both could be correct.

The Cause Of Cavities # 1: Poor Quality Foods

I mentioned Dr. Weston A. Price (1870-1948) earlier. A Cleveland dentist, he observed that the diet of isolated primitive tribes contained at least ten times the amount of fat-soluble vitamins as the standard American diet of his day.

He determined that the abundant presence of fat-soluble Vitamins A and D in their diets, along with other minerals such as calcium and phosphorus, gave the population high immunity to tooth decay and resistance to disease.

Although the 14 tribal diets Dr Price studied over 25 years differed, each of them offered immunity to tooth decay and resistance to disease. These tribal diets included no refined or processed foods and were rich in proteins, minerals, vitamins, and especially in 'fat-soluble factors found in animal fats'.

At least that was until these tribal cultures first integrated with Western civilisation, consuming the "displacing foods of modern commerce." Only then did they begin to show evidence of bone loss, chronic illnesses, tooth decay, and facial deformities (crowded teeth, narrow dental arches, birth defects, and narrow facial structures).

Dr Price also highlighted the lack of Vitamin K in the modern diet. The ingestion of Vitamin K catalyses special proteins that manage the effective distribution of phosphorous and calcium within the teeth. At the same time, it helps reduce internal inflammation by inhibiting calcium from calcifying soft tissues in the kidneys and arteries.

One of Dr. Price's patients was healed of 48 cavities in 24 teeth over a 7-month period using vitamin-rich butter oil.

Dr Prices's conclusion? That the long-term and primary cause of dental decay **IMPORTANT** is mainly nutritional deficiencies.

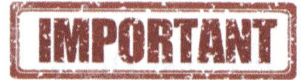

There you have it. The incidence of cavities is linked to what you eat rather than the bacteria in your mouth. For a modern man to have any hope of surviving, the basics of proper nutrition must somehow be re-introduced into today's lifestyle.

As more research is carried out, it's evident that the rogue bacteria in your mouth can cause more damage than you ever thought possible. The secret to keeping a healthy heart and a healthy body may be a healthy mouth.

Yet research results can be confusing. A study in Taiwan (published in the American Journal of Medicine) confirmed that regular dental cleanings decrease the risk of a heart attack or stroke, while another study showed that these cleanings can spread bacteria into the bloodstream if bacterial imbalances, parasites and other 'bad bugs' aren't eliminated before the cleaning.

To underscore Dr Price's work the founders of Loma Linda Dental School, scientists Ralph Steinmann DDS, and John Leonora, PhD (Endocrine Physiology) contributed significantly to the real causes behind tooth decay and evidenced that cavities are not solely caused by bacteria. They were the first scientists to show the existence of a fluid flow between the body and the teeth.

In their slightly more technical speak.....

> *"The parotid hormone is manufactured in the parotid gland (a salivary gland). When produced in adequate amounts (influenced by healthy foods), the resultant fluid flow runs from within the body into the pulp chamber, drawing nutrients to all parts of the tooth, through the dentine, the enamel and into the mouth.*
>
> *When processed or poor quality foods are eaten this fluid flow is reversed. Sludge and bacteria in this instance are dragged from the mouth, into the tooth through the enamel, dentine and pulp where a chemical breakdown takes place. The healthy, outward flow became an unhealthy inward flow simply by altering the diet."*

In other words, you are more prone to cavities when you eat junk food.

A single tooth is made up of many miles of tiny tubuli, which are where nutrients flow. Steinmann and Leonora showed us how tooth decay starts inside the tooth long before any evidence appears on the outside. Sugar makes the body acidic, therefore accelerating tooth decay.

The Cause Of Cavities # 2: Tooth Decay Is An Infection

I've always liked Dr David Kennedy's no-nonsense approach. Speaking on tooth decay he says:

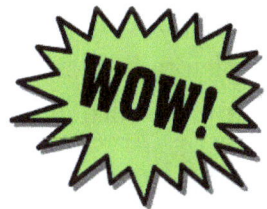

> *"Believe me it's an infection that goes from person to person to person. DNA testing shows it's*

25

coming from the mother or grandmother or the caregiver to the child at about age two.

So it's a germ (Streptococcus Mutans). It's transferred from the people that care for the child. All the germs in the baby's body come from mother. So if there happens to be a bad one in the mix you can very simply get rid of it. You don't need it. It's not a valuable bug. Kill it. So it's gone."

For this, you need to source a broad-spectrum parasite cleanse. Key into YouTube and watch **Bad Bugs (29:12)**. It's information worth knowing and is what today's leading dentists are confirming to their patients.

Repairing Cavities

If a poor diet is the cause of cavities, it stands to reason that improving your diet will not only help reverse cavities but also prevent them from recurring in the future. The internet offers many products that 'heal' cavities.

At best, they may reduce the pain, but that doesn't mean the cavity is repaired - it's just numbed. Unless you want to spend money like a drunken sailor, I'd treat all such offers with suspicion, especially as you now know the best option is to spend your hard-earned money on good food.

Natural Health author and lecturer David Wolfe got it right when he said:

"If something's wrong with our teeth, then something must be wrong with what we're eating."

Dentists usually recommend that any small cavity be filled immediately to avoid greater pain later. In one sense, they're right. What your dentist isn't acknowledging is that teeth are in a constant state of de-mineralisation and re-mineralisation, so decay is not always going to cause greater pain later.

Of course, the best prevention is cutting down on sugar, but try telling the children that, especially at Halloween or their birthday! Sugar is toxic. If you absolutely have to take it, at least do yourself a favour and drop all sugar just before and for a few days after any form of oral surgery, as it will negate the vital recovery process after extraction wounds or implant placements.

The long-standing belief that sugar causes tooth decay carries some weight, but only because it depletes nutrients from the body, not because bacteria devour it to produce acid that wrecks the enamel.

I'll write it again: sugar produces acids that ruin your teeth, BUT it is NOT the source of tooth decay.

I came across introspeck's honest contribution to a blog post:

> *"I've had crappy teeth all my life, too. Until just a few years ago. I basically dropped 95% of the sugar-c containing out of my life. No soda, cookies, candy, anything with sugar. The only exception is ketchup and other sauces, that's the 5%. My teeth and gums are healthy, I haven't gotten cavities, haven't had to pay the dentist for anything."*

I can't put my hand on my heart and write that I have seen this done, but a team of Australian dental researchers at Sydney University conducted a seven-year study that renewed the evidence that dental decay can be reversed.

Professor Wendell Evans concluded that fillings are unnecessary and *"not required in many cases of dental decay"* adding that there is a *"...need for a major shift in the way tooth decay is managed by dentists"*.

To prove that point, a study in adults with active dental decay discovered that half the early tooth lesions found were reversed within 33 months.

The study also concluded that drilling and filling are often unnecessary and *'raise questions about the ethics of continuing this practice."*

David Albert, Associate Professor of Clinical Dentistry at Columbia University, further contributed to the discussion on early decay treatment by suggesting, *"I think we do more harm by over-treating because there will always be complications of treatment"*.

His point was that fillings can crack, break, or fall out, and the space between the filling and the tooth is a hot spot for further decay, which could, in turn, lead to root canal treatment or tooth loss. Drilling weakens the tooth and can threaten neighbouring teeth.

In any case, drilling compromises the strength of the natural tooth arch. Inserting a filling on the chewing side of the tooth damages its structure, weakening the tooth on either side of that filling.

If you still prefer to visit a dentist, you might like to know that new pain-free techniques, such as laser-assisted dentistry and gels, allow cavities to be repaired without drilling or injections.

I'd personally like to know the gel ingredients first. Stem-cell procedures to regrow new teeth in your mouth are also available, although I don't believe they are yet available at any high-street dentist.

Removing Plaque and Tartar

History tells us that Cleopatra VI, beautiful and powerful as she may have been, had such bad calculus that she could physically remove her lower teeth.

Plaque is an invisible material that collects on your teeth every single time you eat or drink. Most of it is removed with sensible hygiene, yet there are places where your toothbrush can't get to it. If words don't make you pay attention, then maybe these images will:

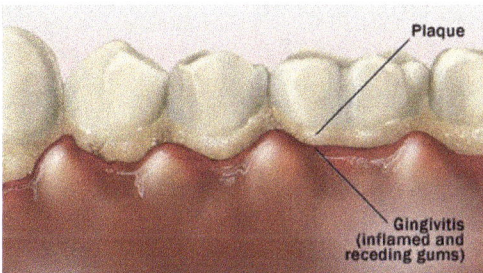

And if you ignore the plaque, it becomes calculus (thanks to Wikipedia for the images)

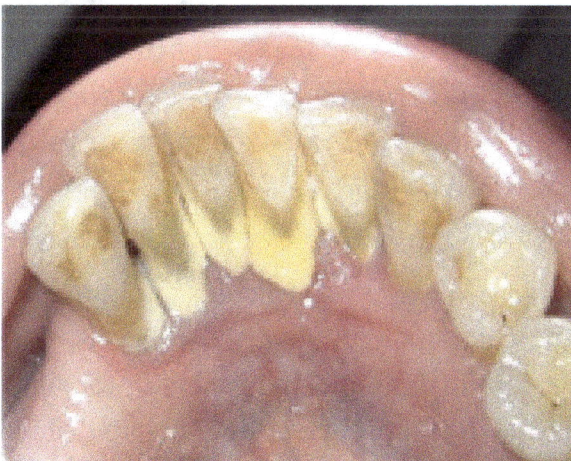

As plaque develops, you'll notice a hard brown-yellowish substance lining the inside of the teeth, especially at the gum line. Plaque contains the bacteria that facilitate gum disease. If you don't take care of it at this stage, the plaque will harden and become calculus (sometimes called tartar).

We think of plaque in terms of the images above and of the plaque itself as colonies of calculus causing all manner of deterioration within the mouth.

Some types of biofilm *protect* our teeth from demineralization

> *"There's an important part of the story is a little known structure called 'dental pellicle'. The pellicle is essentially the beginning biofilm on teeth after cleaning. Formed by proteins from saliva, pellicle is a thin protein layer that coats our teeth. The pellicle provides the 'platform' for oxygen-loving bacteria to attach which begins the lifecycle of a plaque colony. Our culture likes to blame 'bad bugs' as being the cause of tooth decay. And while microbes are part of the story of tooth decay, it's not the whole story. Another major contributor to demineralizing enamel and weakening our teeth is exposing our teeth to acidic foods and drinks."*
>
> Will & Susan, Orawellness

The consequences of ignoring calculus build-up could include diabetes, cancer and a lengthy list of conditions you really don't want to have. Scientists found that bacteria-causing plaque can invade the part of your immune system responsible for attacking cancer cells, interfering with their protective role.

The British Medical Journal Open (2012) reported researchers at University of Helsinki confirming that people with high levels of dental plaque were 80% more likely to die prematurely of cancer than people with little plaque.

Back as far as 1833, Surgeon-Dentist John Nicholles, in his book 'The Teeth in Relation to Beauty, Voice and Health' wrote...

"The tendency of tartar is to separate the teeth from the gums, to loosen them in their sockets, to irritate the contiguous parts, and to produce inflammation. The tendency of the accumulation of particles of food is to undergo the putrefactive process, to act upon the enamel and to penetrate the bone, causing toothache and destroying the teeth. Nor does the evil rest here; diseases of these parts, like all other local affections produce derangements of the various bodily functions. Simple caries of the teeth will sometimes give rise to what the French have called tic douloureux* to disorders of the ear, of the stomach and other organs; it has even been known to set up excruciating pain in the limbs analogous to rheumatism."

* tic douloureux, though exceedingly painful, is nothing more than the irritation of certain nerves of the face, and in most cases proceeds originally from the teeth.

Any plaque forming overnight should be removed in the morning. This can be done in several ways, and success, of course, depends on your diligence. If left to harden from plaque into tartar, an overload of bacteria may then travel throughout your bloodstream.

Natural Ways To Remove Plaque From Your Teeth

We're in the 21st century, a very advanced technological age. These may seem like old methods used but they're here because they contribute to the removal of plaque.

- Place some unrefined sea salt on a damp, clean cloth. Begin gently rubbing this salt onto your teeth inside and out, especially where your teeth meet the gums. Rinse with water.
- Mix a teaspoon of bicarbonate of soda with a pinch of unrefined sea salt and about 1 1/2 teaspoons of coconut oil. Adding a dash of Manuka Honey improves the result. Combine all the ingredients together and apply the mix to your teeth first by rinsing around your mouth, followed by a thorough brushing as you spit out. Rinse your mouth with water afterwards.
- Mix a tablespoon of apple cider vinegar with 2 tablespoons of water. Rinse the mixture around your mouth vigorously for 2-3 minutes. Spit it out and then rinse it with water, as apple cider vinegar is highly acidic.

If you want evidence of these recommendations working, buy a plaque marking solution to identify plaque locations in your mouth before starting.

Toothache

There are few agonies in life so persistent, so maddeningly relentless, as the dull throb of an angry tooth. I've been fortunate, if you can call it that, to have experienced this uniquely sadistic torment only once - from a dying tooth.

It's an excruciating pain I never want to go through again.

Nothing relieves the constant pulsating; you can't sleep, and the programmes on TV at 2 am are usually appalling.

It feels as though your whole jawbone is on fire and the intense, throbbing pain seems to be in rhythm with your pulse. Toothache mostly occurs on the Friday evening of a Bank Holiday weekend when your dentist has gone fishing.

As with all symptoms, an aching tooth is often the body's way of telling you of a more serious problem elsewhere.

Toothache can be tricky, especially if you're unsure what's causing the pain. Pain is not always a reliable indicator of what's really going on. While many toothaches are caused by tooth decay, pain is also caused by a cracked tooth, an abscess or an impacted wisdom tooth. Even gum disease can bring about intense pain, often mistaken as toothache.

These are worth looking at if you're waiting for that appointment with your dentist.

Key into your YouTube or your browser and watch:

Acupressure Points For Toothache (1:45)

10 Soothing Acupressure Points to Relieve Toothache

Toothache Remedies

Cloves are a consistently recommended folk remedy. Containing eugenol, a natural analgesic used by dentists to kill germs and alleviate gum pain, cloves are definitely one for your dental first-aid kit. I prefer to suck on a whole clove. If there's no other choice, mix half a teaspoon of coconut oil with 2 or 3 drops of clove oil on a cotton ball and pack it against the area of pain for as long as you consider appropriate. Be sure to rinse your mouth with water afterwards.

Cayenne and Ginger: Mix diced ginger and cayenne (and a little water) to create a paste. To help reduce the pain and swelling, apply the paste directly using a cotton ball (or cotton tip).

Garlic has many beneficial properties, including the ability to fight bacteria and viruses. Raw garlic is best for this. Crush a clove of garlic and add a pinch of unrefined sea salt before applying it to the painful area.

Many years ago, I was involved in a project with Peter Josling, director of the Garlic Centre in Sussex, England. What Peter didn't know about garlic wasn't worth knowing. He agreed that people with a toothache should either chew a raw clove near the infected tooth or crush a garlic clove and place it around the tooth.

Peppermint has been a popular toothache-relieving potion with antiseptic properties. If you are in pain, make a brew of hot water and peppermint leaves.

Ice: Apply an ice cube or ice pack directly to the painful area or to the external cheek. Alternatively, you can address the pain through a reflex action such as immersing your body in cold water or walking barefoot in snow. Apply an ice cube to the shoulder on the same side as the pain.

Homeopathic Remedies Contact a qualified homoeopath for more details. Chamomile or Belladonna are often recommended to be taken every 15 minutes until you see a dentist.

Pressure Points: apply pressure to the hand on the affected side, at the fleshy area where the base of the index finger and the thumb meet. Even holding this "Hoku" point for a few minutes will release pain-relieving endorphins.

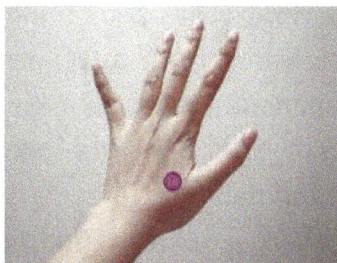

One of the most helpful charts I have used is the **Pointfinder Pain Chart** on pointfinder.org

Tooth Grinding (Bruxism)
Tooth grinding is a habit that may not at first appear serious, but in the long term, it can cause a range of debilitating conditions in your teeth and gums. Doctors and dentists have yet to determine the cause of tooth grinding. One theory suggested that tooth grinding was stress-related, but this suggestion didn't explain why foetuses were observed tooth grinding in utero.

In addition to the studies that indicate the lack of breastfeeding in infancy as a primary cause, a new theory has shed some light on the cause....parasites.

Parasites: Hells Angels Of The Blood Stream

I've heard some people claiming that parasites only affect the gut. Others have a mistaken belief that there are 'good' parasites and 'bad' parasites. One English doctor flatly refused to accept the fact that parasites existed in the UK. *'Poppycock! This is Britain,"* he uttered as he showed me the way out of his clinic.

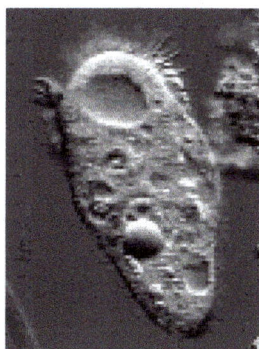

Several years ago, I thought I'd learn something useful about parasites from an experienced vet practising in the South of England. As I spoke, he asked, *"In which animals?"* I replied, *"I'm talking about parasites found in humans rather than animals."* His demeanour changed abruptly as he declared, *"There is no such thing as a parasite in the human being"*. His experience had been entirely with animals. He was clearly embarrassed that hadn't been taught about parasites in humans, and therefore, to him, they didn't exist. He certainly didn't want to learn about them from me.

Eat a cubic inch of prime, grade A, organic beef, and you'll ingest anything up to 1000 parasite larvae. Shaking hands, drinking tap water, eating undercooked foods, changing nappies, kissing partners and friends.....all contribute to a level of parasitic transfer.

Parasites have been the biggest killer of mankind since the Stone Age. They are rarely, if ever, listed on death certificates or shown as a cause of death league tables because of their ability to mimic the symptoms of more common diseases. From microscopic protozoa to a 60ft tapeworm, your body's ability to handle and reject parasites is what determines your lifetime health.

Appalling as it may seem, tooth grinding (bruxism) has been identified as a symptom of pinworms (Enterobius vermicularis), roundworms (Ascaris lumbricoides), and other intestinal parasites. The mistaken belief that parasites only inhabit the gut is far from accurate, as parasites can be found under the fingernails, in the eyeball, and in the bloodstream, from where they can travel anywhere in the body.

Dr Dietrich Klinghardt, a world-renowned specialist in neuro-toxins and parasitic diseases, writes (translated from the original German).

"The parasite issue is one of the most overlooked issues in the world today. It is known that the reason we have better longevity now than we had a hundred years ago is not attributable to any of the medical advances – antibiotics, operations, cardiac bypass surgery, none of that – it's only attributable to advances in hygiene that we have made. There is enough evidence to say that whether we live long and are healthy or not is not any of the other aspects of medicine, but how we deal with parasites. One area that we address in medicine quite a bit is a thing called bone cavitations in the jaw bone. This is usually when teeth go bad in the mouth, or they die then are extracted, the jaw bone very often stays behind infected. The Germans have found that people that have roundworms and tapeworms very frequently lost teeth – teeth simply start dying at the root, then often get extracted or they stay in there and the jawbone gets infected in the area. That is caused by a toxin release from the worms in the gut. The toxins are then absorbed and has this effect on the teeth which are very sensitive structures. Completely unrelated on the surface but intrinsically very much related to the worm infestation. Intrinsic toxins are created in the gut by parasites and are then absorbed causing dysfunctions in the bio- chemistry leading to chronic tiredness. When people wake up in the morning and they don't feel fresh and rested very often this is a symptom of chronic parasites in the gut or elsewhere. The worm called Ascaris

Lumbricoides (Roundworm) which is the most common worm that I find in people gives off a poison that's called Ascaradine, one of the most studied toxins from worms which has exactly that effect."

His point? The state of your gum health can be directly related to the parasitic activity in your gut. Concerned? Ask your dentist if there are facilities to check your oral biofilm with a microscope. Some worms are too microscopic to be picked up by a standard microscope in which case a more thorough parasite testing can be undertaken by a diagnostic parasite laboratory.

Missing Teeth

A 2017 study published in the Journal of the American Geriatrics Society has confirmed the link between missing teeth and Alzheimer's disease. 'Missing' teeth include teeth that have been violently knocked out in a boxing match or car accident, as well as teeth removed by a dentist.

Toothpastes: What To Beware Of

Most toothpastes are not as good as we are led to believe as they contain glycerin. This coats and remains on the teeth thus blocking the naturally-occurring remineralisation process. Your saliva strengthens the enamel but can't do its job when teeth are coated in glycerine.

The first thing to look for in the toothpaste you're currently using is the presence of tiny microbeads. Made from plastic specks of polyethylene, these beads remain in your mouth after rinsing.

When spat out into the basin, they are washed into the sea, where they are consumed by marine life, with consequences.

It doesn't end there. Fish are caught, and they end up on your dinner plate, where you consume the microplastic all over again.

In 2014, Proctor & Gamble (Crest) asserted that the ingredients in its toothpaste were safe. I wondered what form of Columbian inhalation therapy were their advisors were on when they came up with that claim. Subsequently, P & G agreed to remove all polyethylene microbeads by 2016 because of a *'growing consumer preference."*

My questions are:

- why did they even think of adding polyethylene in the first place?
- once discovered, why did they take so long to remove the microbeads?

Anyone using this toothpaste up until 2016 should be aware of what they've been putting in their mouth. "Safe?" There's a growing difference between "safe" and "FDA safe".

Be in no doubt as to what toothpaste really is - a mixture of ingredients that act as a chemical anaesthetic to your teeth and gums. Look at the ingredients. You'll see that many brands contain fluoride and other toxic additives you really shouldn't have in your mouth. Read on and you'll see that they do us more harm than good.

First thing to look for is the distinct colour on the tube:

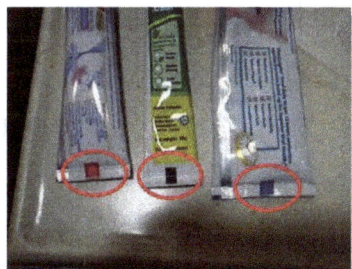

Green = 'Natural'
Blue = Natural plus medicinal compounds.

Red = Natural + some form of Chemical composition.

Black = Pure Chemical

Don't believe me? If too much toothpaste is swallowed by a child in a day it could result in fluoride poisoning and/or mottling of the tooth enamel. So the FDA warns people about the potential harm caused by toothpaste and people still use it!

> The food and Drug Administration (USA) requires, as of April 1997 that all fluoride-containing toothpaste and mouth rinse carry a poison label, warning that the products be kept out of reach of children under 6, and to contact a Poison Control Centre if more than the amount for brushing (pea-sized drop) is swallowed.

Reminds me of the saying, "*Everything is hidden in plain sight*".

The FDA compounds the issue by telling you that only a pea-sized drop is enough! Call me crazy, but any amount of fluoride is not something you want to put in your mouth. So why do we do it? It's called 'conditioning,' and we've all fallen for it at some point.

People think they need to smear toothpaste along the entire length of the bristles. Why? Because the advertising shows this. Dentists agree the pea-sized drop is quite sufficient. Your toothpaste will last much longer!

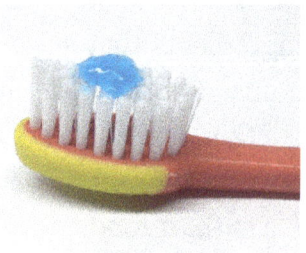

The FDA has approved toothpastes that claim on the label '*to prevent gingivitis and plaque,"* but you may not be that keen on having questionable pharmaceuticals in your body without good reason.

TV commercials usually show actors with photoshopped white teeth smiling as they brush. There's usually a little foaming, and after 15 seconds or so, they smile at the camera with their sparkly clean teeth.

Remember, it's just an ad. Behind the scenes, all is not as we think. Let's go through a few of the Triple-X-Avoid ingredients that make up many toothpastes:

- **Sodium Lauryl Sulfate** creates the foaming effect. It's a toxin and may cause neurological damage as well as damage to human tissue (skin irritant), reproductive activity and internal organs. Spit SLS into the basin, it then pollutes the rivers and seas, where the harm continues to aquatic creatures. What's ironic is that SLS may well cause periodontitis....and periodontitis is what you're reading this ebook to avoid!

Slippery as always, manufacturers now claim that the SLS used is 'derived from coconuts'. Someone's speaking with a forked tongue! What they fail to mention is that the SLS is then mixed together with an assortment of harsh chemicals that should be avoided individually and collectively.

Pinocchio has nothing on these guys.

- **Fluoride** is heavily promoted as preventing tooth decay.....but it doesn't do this. It has even been added to the public water supply and reservoirs in many areas. There is simply no excuse to add fluoride to oral care products or drinking water. Anywhere.
- **Triclosan:** In September 2016 the FDA banned the anti-bacterial agent triclosan used in detergents, soaps, cosmetics, toys and toothpaste. Despite hundreds of positive research studies submitted (be suspicious of any

'independent' research these days!), the Natural Resource Defense Council said of triclosan in a statement, " *For starters, it's an endocrine disruptor, meaning it interferes with important hormone functions, which can directly affect the brain in addition to our immune and reproductive systems.*"

- **Food colouring dyes** are a by-product of coal tar and petroleum and have been linked to behavioural problems.
- **Carrageenan** (aka Irish Moss): Food-grade carrageenan can induce gastrointestinal inflammation, ulcerations and lesions. And for those deranged people who test nasty products on animals, it has also been shown to cause colon cancer in laboratory animals.
- **Hydrated Silica** is a harsh abrasive whitener derived from sand. This is not what you want as it can destroy your tooth enamel.
- **Sweeteners:** Artificial sweeteners such as aspartame are toxic. Cooking with them or having them with your tea/coffee is already damaging your health. Adding artificial sweeteners to toothpaste just isn't necessary.

The PR departments, of course come up with their carefully worded soundbite phrases like:

"Years of clinical research show no evidence of (whatever the ingredient they're promoting) causing any harm", and....

"We are not immediately aware of any safety issues with this product."

The use of the words *"no evidence"* and *"immediately aware"* are sleight-of-mouth. They're lying like flatfish, so get into the habit of making your own toothpaste. You'll realise how straight-forward it is once you've done it a couple of times.

...or pop into your local health food store, where you'll find some good fluoride-free toothpastes. Be sure to READ THOSE LABELS for other suspicious ingredients, especially the ones you can't pronounce.

Home Made Toothpaste

With its wide range of health benefits, including antibacterial and antifungal properties, coconut oil is the perfect base for homemade toothpaste. It helps to kill harmful bacteria (including Streptococcus Mutans and Candida Albicans) in your mouth as you brush.

- **basic mix** The simplest method to make your own toothpaste at home is by mixing 4 tablespoons of coconut oil with 5 tablespoons of bicarbonate of soda. When that's mixed into a paste, add 10-15 trace mineral drops, which you can buy online or in most health food stores. To improve on these basic ingredients, you can add:
  - 1 tablespoon of bentonite clay (optional but improves the effectiveness)
  - several drops of stevia (better than Xylitol) to offset any mild bitterness
  - a teaspoon of Activated Charcoal
  - crushed cacao nibs

- Cacao - the ideal toothpaste would be a cacao toothpaste since compounds in cacao beans promote remineralisation better than fluoride (and, of course, much more safely). Depending on the grain size of the cacao nibs, breaking up the biofilm could be a safe abrasive — just like ground walnut shells are used to polish jewellery!

- Bicarbonate of soda - for its alkalinity. Thanks to the foods we eat, Our mouths are constantly under attack by acids, Neutralising these acids with vegetables and water is essential to maintaining proper pH in the mouth to encourage the right bacteria and protect enamel from decay. It has an alkaline pH, so it helps neutralise acids while not being too abrasive for teeth.

Get used to the basic ingredients and then start to experiment with ingredients like coconut oil, activated charcoal, myrrh gum powder.....

Despite the Pharma-funded studies telling us how bad coconut oil is, it is your best friend.

Some people are concerned that coconut oil will clog drains. If this is a concern, just spit the toothpaste in a disposal bin or onto the grass outside when you're finished.

- *chocolate (cacao) toothpaste*

Here's the best chocolate (cacao) toothpaste recipe to make yourself:

Ingredients

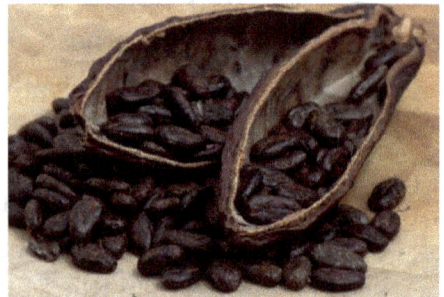

- 2 tablespoons bicarbonate of soda
- 4 tablespoons coconut oil
- 3-4 drops peppermint extract
- 2 teaspoons cacao powder
- unrefined sea salt

Directions

1. Mix the bicarbonate of soda, cacao powder and unrefined sea salt together
2. Add peppermint extract and slightly warmed coconut oil, stirring well
3. Keep in a sealed jar or other sealed container.
4. Scoop a pea-sized amount out with a spoon and place on the bristles of your brush

- ***activated charcoal toothpaste***

Ingredients

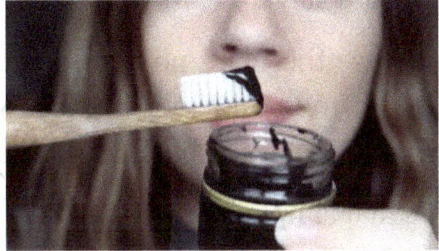

- 1/2 cup bicarbonate of soda
- 2 teaspoon of activated charcoal
- 2 teaspoon of coconut oil
- unrefined sea salt
- 8-10 drops peppermint extract

Directions

1. Mix the bicarbonate of soda, activated charcoal and unrefined sea salt together
2. Add the peppermint extract and slightly warmed coconut oil, stirring well
3. Keep in a sealed jar or other sealed container
4. Scoop a pea-sized amount out with a spoon and place on the bristles of your brush

Now you can see how easy it is to make basic toothpaste at home. Here's another simple recipe I found that differs slightly in terms of ingredients and directions but it'll be just as effective. Note the essential oil is food grade.

Key into YouTube and watch any video on **Activated Charcoal Toothpaste**

- ***remineralising toothpaste***
  - mix 5 teaspoons of calcium carbonate powder with 1 teaspoon Diatomaceous Earth
  - Add 1 teaspoon bicarbonate of soda and 3 teaspoons coconut oil. Mix well.
  - Add stevia to taste

Because there are no ingredients in the toothpaste that will go bad so-to-speak, this product will keep for a long time, but making it in small batches is best.

It's that simple.

Toothbrushes

Look at the display of toothbrushes arranged on a supermarket shelf and there's a commonality. Most people choose according to price or colour. Some brushes have raised thumb mounds, others have varying-height bristle rows and many display go-faster stripes. You're forgiven for not knowing what's best for you. Personally I don't buy any of these, preferring the brushes with wooden or bamboo handles available online or at a health food store.

It is difficult to find a toothbrush that is wholly biodegradable. Many toothbrush manufacturers that claim their bristles are degradable, being made from Nylon-4 (ask to see the proof) but they are really made from Nylon-6. Nylon-6 is not biodegradable.

Bamboo Brushes

Ecological bamboo toothbrushes should have BPA free, soft bristles (hard bristles can damage sensitive gums) and with luck even the box and brush wrapper will be recyclable. Bamboo is one if the fastest growing sustainable plants on the earth and there are so many wonderful initiatives, including bamboo architecture.

Two billion plastic brushes are dumped into landfill annually. Every purchase of a bamboo toothbrush is a vote against plastic and helps bring about fresh ecological initiatives.

Blotting Brushes & MiniBlots

In terms of effectiveness, Blotting Brushes and the smaller-headed MiniBlots (for children) put all other toothbrushes I've ever come across to shame. Originally designed in the 1960s by Dr. Joseph Phillips, an international figure in oral health (at one point teaching dental surgery at UCLA), for many, these brushes were a saviour to their dental health.

I started using the Blotting Brushes in 2001. To me, they were undoubtedly the *bee's knees* of toothbrushes, one bonus being that no toothpaste was ever required on the bristles.

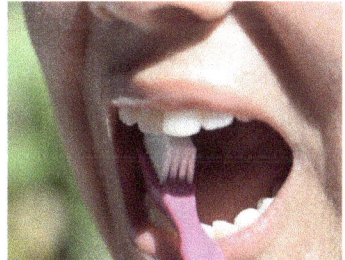

For first-time users, I would suggest they clean their teeth at night using a conventional brush and toothpaste. When finished, use their Blotting Brush. They were always surprised by the particles of food and oral debris that would subsequently be dislodged.

Unfortunately, the company that manufactured the Blotting Brushes and MiniBlots terminated production during lockdown without giving us any notice. Thanks to the support from Dr. Phillips' family members, I now have useful guidelines on how the bristles are treated before they are affixed to the handle.

In the 15 years between 2005 (when we first started offering them) and 2020 (when production was terminated), we had only three requests for a refund. Two elderly ladies suffering from degenerative neurological conditions that couldn't manage the technique. The third was from a customer wanting his money back after only a few days. He did admit to wanting something that would resolve the poor condition of his mouth without him having to do much!

The biggest problem we've faced has been finding a toothbrush manufacturer prepared to take on board a range of boutique brushes. We've tried several but they could never get the particulars right, always hoping we would accept their version.

Until we find a new manufacturer the absence of the Blotting Brushes and MiniBlots is a great loss to the world of dental health.

If you'd like to be alerted about the arrival of stocks of these brushes when and if we can have them replicated, register yourself for our weekly newsletter on a wide range of natural health issues and we'll let you know.

Newsletter site: *www.resourcesforlife.net* (scroll to the foot of the website page to register)

1. Place the brush at an angle against the tooth, making certain that the bristles are at the gumline. Gently brush the surface of each tooth using a short, gentle vibrating motion.

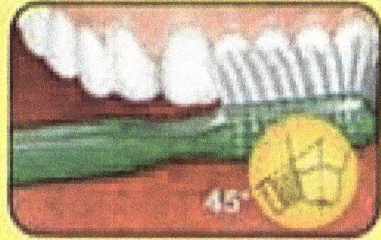

2. Brush the outer surfaces of each tooth, upper and lower, keeping the bristles angled against the gumline. Repeat the same method on the inner surfaces of the teeth as well.

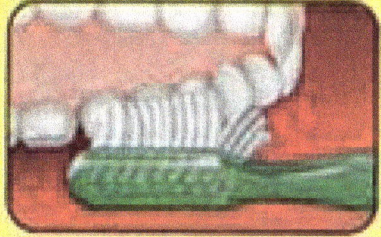

3. To clean the inside surfaces of the front teeth, tilt the brush vertically and make several gentle up-and-down strokes using the front half of the brush.

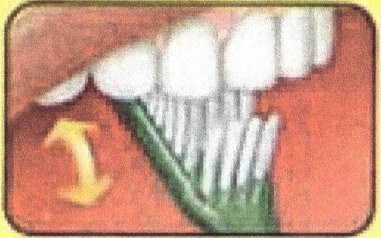

4. Scrub the chewing surfaces of the teeth using a short back and forth movement. Brushing the tongue will remove bacteria and freshen your breath.

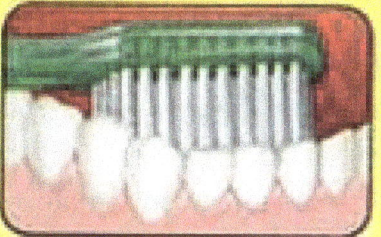

Bass Brushes

Dr. Charles Bass developed the Bass Brushing method, probably because his gum disease was advanced and his teeth were threatening to fall out. That was the trigger for him. On being told a complete removal of his teeth was next, he set to work to restore his gum health.

Using the microscope, Dr. Bass determined which strains of bacteria were doing the damage. Eventually identifying a method of brushing that reversed his condition, it is believed that he died with all his teeth intact.

While the Bass Brushes are recommended for this method some people have observed benefits from using this method with their regular toothbrushes.

Whichever method you use, you should brush your teeth BEFORE meals.

Professor Mike Edgar, University of Newcastle told the International Dental Conference On Caries Research *"Brushing teeth after eating is a bit like shutting the gate after the horse has bolted"*, adding *"acid production after eating is very rapid."*

Dental Water Jets

People ask me about using dental water jets or oral irrigators. If used sensibly, they are better than flossing. However, one particular value they provide is eliminating BUGS from the enamel on your teeth and gums. More and more dentists are recommending dental water jets as a flossing alternative.

The technique uses a jet of pressurised water to clean between the teeth and the gum line.

Theoretically, these water jets remove bacteria in deep periodontal pockets that can't be reached through brushing or flossing.

I'll repeat here that I'm in favour of anything encouraging people to clean their teeth and gums, but there's a double bind here. A high water speed setting is required to remove debris and plaque from the gum pockets. The problem with a high water speed setting is that the elasticity of the gumline may be damaged, allowing more plaque and other debris into the pocket.

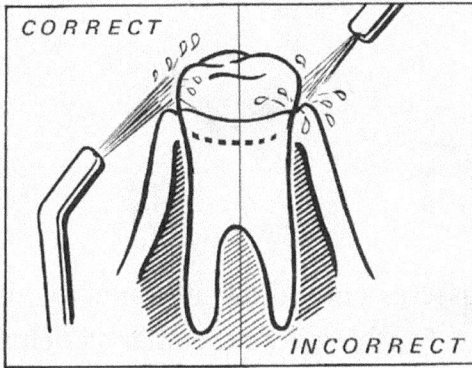

Figure 37. Correct & incorrect way of directing irrigating device.

The only solution I can make is to direct the water, as shown in the image.

Neem/Mustard Tree Sticks

Miswak is the root of the "Peelu" tree (Salvadora Persica), known in the Middle East as the Arak Tree. The miswak stick has been used for centuries in Middle Eastern & African societies to suppress decay, gingivitis and plaque formation.

Scientific research confirms its antibacterial and plaque-fighting properties, and the World Health Organization has recommended it for its dental hygiene benefits.

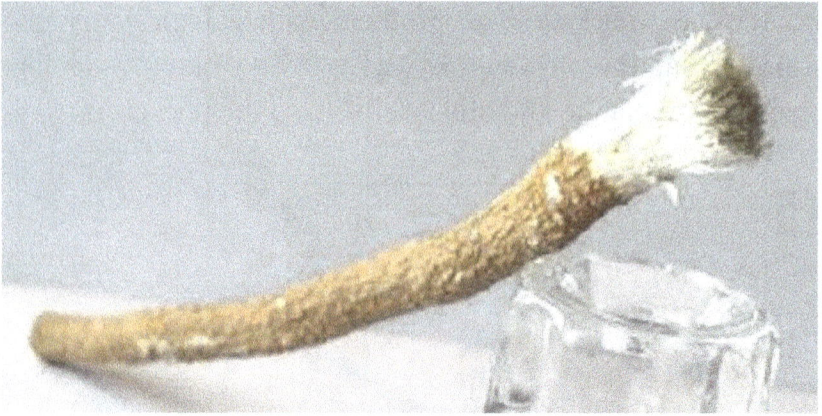

The miswak possesses natural disinfectants that clean teeth and strengthen gums. Brushing with the miswak helps eliminate bad breath and improves taste buds. No toothpaste is required.

Tooth Cleaning Gadgets

I've seen ads for gadgets that claim to clean or whiten teeth in seconds. I'm happy when there's any form of encouragement to remove food and other debris from the mouth, but I don't hold out any hope with most of the gadgets being marketed, as dental health isn't about speed or having shiny white teeth.

The whole mouth needs proper attention, which doesn't happen in 10 seconds. Gadgets may be useful for people with debilitating conditions such as Parkinson's Disease. Try one if you like, but I reckon you'll be back in the dentist's chair quicker than a New York minute.

Teeth Whitening: Avoid Short-Term Solutions For Long-Term Conditions

Hollywood celebrities seem to have perfect whitened teeth. It's probably a casting requirement. The celebrity culture some people mindlessly follow has made white teeth into a must-have cosmetic treatment.

The whitening process, if carried out by inexperienced people, can lead to permanent damage, so be careful. Read that last sentence again as I used the words 'permanent damage'. Mouth guards containing a gel impregnated with hydrogen peroxide and chemicals are usually fitted into the mouth and left for a short time while the ingredients whiten the teeth.

What could possibly go wrong?

For starters, the bleaching gel can leak from the mouth guard and either be swallowed (inducing vomiting) or cause chemical burns to the gums.

I'll write it again - "White" teeth do not necessarily mean "healthy" teeth. Bleaching your teeth is dangerous, can be expensive, and will in time strip enamel away. Instead, there are several options, although they will be slower than a chemical blast to your enamel.

I won't give specific quantities here because they tend to vary when I make the concoction. I would, however, suggest that when making anything with hydrogen peroxide, err on the side of caution.

I use diluted food-grade hydrogen peroxide from time to time, but always with considerable caution. Dentists can perform teeth whitening sessions, but not beauticians. It's all about training.

Home whitening kits can be legally purchased, although they contain only 0.1% hydrogen peroxide, which is barely effective.

Scour the internet for natural tooth-whitening solutions, and you'll be presented with websites that sing the praises of coconut oil as a tooth whitener. Coconut oil has many health benefits, although, in my experience, it takes two to three months of oil pulling to achieve the whiteness you see on the before-and-after website images. That shouldn't matter, as good health is a long-term mission.

- oil pulling is swishing coconut (or other) oil around your mouth for 15-20 minutes each day. Mornings are best. It seems to be the most recommended method, with websites displaying impressive before-and-after images of teeth that have been whitened this way. To benefit from coconut oil's many remedial attributes, in the mornings, I swish half a teaspoon of it around my mouth for 15 - 20 minutes. At night I swallow 2 tablespoons of coconut oil.

To 'oil pull', swish a teaspoon of coconut oil around your mouth, forcing it between your teeth and remembering to reach those far upper and lower reaches. It will mix with your saliva. When finished, spit it out somewhere that won't clog up the water pipes. Spit it out. Rinse your mouth with warm water afterwards. If, for any reason, you experience a detox reaction (headaches, flu-like symptoms), stop for a few days and restart when you feel the time is appropriate. Use common sense.

Coconut oil has benefitted people's lives in many ways - eliminating plaque, healing gums, stopping gum bleeding, sleeping better, fresher breath, improving skin and feeling much more energised.

- lemon juice and bicarbonate of soda. Squeeze half a lemon and add half a teaspoon of bicarbonate of soda. It'll fizz up right away. If it's too concentrated, add some water. Swish it around your mouth for as long as possible, remembering to force it between your teeth. I do this once a week at most. Lemon juice is great for stimulating the re-growth of receding gums but is acidic and used excessively to damage tooth enamel. Once inside your body, lemon juice becomes alkaline.

- activated charcoal pulls toxins and teeth-staining tannins from your mouth. Add a teaspoon of activated charcoal into a glass before adding a small amount of water. Stir and rinse around your mouth for a few minutes. Brush your teeth as you spit it out. Activated charcoal is great. Activated bamboo charcoal is even better. Clean up the mess afterwards!

- 35% food grade hydrogen peroxide diluted to 3%, Be extremely careful here to dilute the H_2O_2 to 3% before use. I've included H_2O_2 here because everyone will expect to see it listed. Nevertheless, I include a warning that if you're using it for whitening teeth, it should be in contact with tooth enamel for longer than it would when used as a mouthwash or toothpaste. Being highly acidic, you also want to keep H_2O_2 away from the soft tissues of your mouth. H_2O_2 is manufactured in concentrations of 35% and 50%. The words "food grade" are only a government assurance that it is safe for human consumption. In my experience, all other concentrations (3%, 8% and 12%) that claim to be food grade contain health-destroying

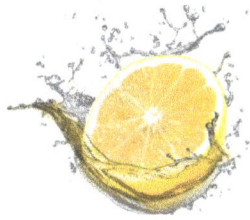

'fillers' - heavy metals, chemical additives and stabilisers. Be careful not to use these or the H2O2 sold from beauty salons, as these are not for oral use. For some reason many governments have restricted the purchase of 35% food grade hydrogen peroxide.

- apple cider vinegar (ACV) and bicarbonate of soda Mix as above for lemon juice and bicarbonate of soda. ACV is highly acidic, so use with discretion and rinse with water when finished

- MMS (Miracle Mineral Solution aka Master Mineral Solution) is a chemical oxidiser that mixes with water, killing pathogen-causing diseases without touching anything else. MMS destroys many poisons and heavy metal compounds in the water.

When activated with Citric Acid, MMS becomes a ruthless destroyer of pathogens. Known as Chlorine Dioxide (CIO2), this is NOT chlorine. Chlorine Dioxide has been sold in chemical form to purify water as sodium chlorite or stabilised oxygen and is one of the most effective killers of pathogens, viruses, moulds, parasites, and other disease-causing organisms known to man.

No gas, powerful industrial acids, pesticides, or other chemical kills pathogens better than chlorine dioxide. It is one of the few things that can even kill anthrax. It can also be used with caution as a tooth whitener.

- Strawberries, oranges, carrot ends and banana peels: Next time you cut up strawberries or peel an orangem cut the end off a carrot or banana, rub the peel against your teeth. Use organic fruit to avoid coating your teeth with unwanted chemicals.

To help any plaque soften, let the film sit on your teeth for a few minutes.

Part Three:

Gum Disease - The Last Frontier

A report from the Singapore Government showed that 85% of Singaporeans have gum disease, attributed to a low incidence of breastfeeding. Feeding from the breast develops the orbicular muscle of the mouth; this is not the case with bottle feeding, where considerably less sucking is required. When bottle-fed children become adults, their weaker orbicular muscles often cause them to sleep and breathe with an open mouth.

Why The Fuss About Bacteria Then?

The first thing to know is that there really are no "good" and "bad" bacteria. Our mouths are full of bacteria, and we should manage the delicate balance rather than eliminate it. When bacteria are considered "bad," they become out of balance with each other, and one type of bacteria, such as Streptococcus mutans, dominates.

That's when we need to redress the imbalance. From here on I'll refer to what we term 'bad' bacteria as 'rogue' bacteria.

"It is interesting to note how the forestry department's idea of sterilizing the soil before seeding trees backfired. They had the belief that if trees were seeded in sterile soil, the seedlings would go free of disease; but, instead, when disease producing bacteria found their way into the seedbeds, there were no good bacteria to counterbalance their growth.

The surest and safest way to have health is to encourage beneficial bacteria to keep the disease-forming bacteria in control. A clean mouth encourages the growth of the health- producing bacteria and, at the same time, limits their activity so that the bacteria cannot go under the crevice where they are not wanted. When experiments were done to count the number of bacteria in the mouth, it was found that the cleaner the mouth, the greater the number of beneficial bacteria present. In many cases, the clean mouth had nearly ten times more bacteria than the dirty one. As one biologist explained, such a condition existed because a greater number of different strains could live in the clean environment, while fewer could exist when the mouth was unclean."

Rogue bacteria take advantage of whatever opportunities they're given, especially in an acidic environment where they can wreak havoc. New strains appear and any reliance on questionable modern medicines is risky when so many natural remedies have already proven effective.

Remove the acidity from your mouth, and bacteria will become less of a problem.

Bacteria build up in your mouth overnight. It makes sense to brush and use a tongue scraper *before* breakfast. This can help freshen your breath and remove any plaque that developed overnight.

Tooth decay affects the enamel and the dentine (inner layer). Bacteria can worsen things, especially when the residue of carbohydrate foods stays on unbrushed teeth. Bacteria live happily within plaque.

Tooth regeneration is quite possible and surprisingly easy. We're told that when tooth decay sets in, it's impossible to reverse. But what may have been impossible yesterday becomes possible today, so read on, and you'll find several ways to help you reverse cavities.

Many people swear by healing cavities using eggshells. I've not tried this myself but the concept appears with reasonable frequency across social media.

Looking at things differently, In 1919, Henry Percy Pickerill concluded:

> *"Bacterial plaques upon the teeth are not an essential factor in the causation of caries, and that the lodgement and infection of carbohydrate material is the essential factor and that those circumstances which favour the formation of bacterial plaques upon the teeth also favour the lodgement of carbohydrates and so the occurrence of the two usually coincides."*

That's a long-winded way of telling you that cavities are caused by carbohydrate foods rather than bacteria.

Pathogenic Bacteria And The Lurking Dangers.....

Streptococcus Mutans are among the potentially harmful rogue bacteria in your mouth. Considered to be the most cariogenic (causing tooth decay) of all of the oral streptococci (there are streptococci cousins!), it sticks to the surface of your teeth and lives off the breads, pasta, potatoes, rice and other carbohydrates you eat. Bacteria convert sugar and starch into acids.

While metabolising sugar and other energy sources, Streptococcus Mutans produce an acid that can cause your tooth enamel to dissolve, accelerating any decay. These acids break down the solid outer surface of your teeth and expose the unprotected, much softer, vulnerable areas – the dentine. As your tooth decays, the nerve (pulp) inside can become infected, bringing with it pain and the likelihood of an abscess.

Disease-causing bacteria flourish and multiply in pockets under your gums. A pocket, just as it sounds, is a space between your gum and your tooth. You may not know these pockets exist, but years of plaque cause your gum lines to slowly pull away from your teeth and form these spaces.

Providing a warm, oxygen-free, nutrient-rich environment makes these pockets an ideal breeding ground for pathogenic bacteria to grow and reproduce. If allowed to grow out of control, these pathogenic bacteria or their toxic waste products enter your bloodstream, are transported through the body and can cause infection.

You need to be careful here. Bacterial infection can bring about a state of chronic inflammation in your blood. Chronic inflammation of any sort leads to chronic disease. Failing to take care of your teeth may set you up for a range of serious medical issues such as heart disease, diabetes, pre-term birth delivery, and Alzheimer's and can even promote cancers,

The presence of bacteria does not necessarily mean there is an infection. Signs of swelling, bleeding, redness, and pus are clear signs of infection. At this early stage, pain is not necessarily a symptom. If you suffer from this, I'd suggest you make an appointment to see your hygienist or dentist. It is difficult to eliminate bacteria from these pockets with a high-pressure water flosser without destroying filaments.

Gum Disease - The Hidden Dangers

The first symptom of gum disease is swollen gums. You'll probably see some blood coming from your gums when you brush your teeth; other times, your gums may feel sensitive or sore. This can be accompanied by unusual tastes or even bad breath.

When chewing becomes painful, a tooth may have loosened, or the gums may have visibly separated from the teeth. If this is the case, you have gum disease or possibly periodontitis. This is serious, and you need to speak with your dentist.

Let's look at what may be the most likely causes.

- look at how often you clean your teeth and for how long
- has your tongue been pierced?
- do you brush your teeth like a crazed ferret on steroids or do you brush them gently? The perception that 'harder is

better' when it comes to tooth brushing is completely and utterly the wrong thing to do.

If you didn't raise your hand to any of the above, it could be something you might want to blame on your genes. We've been programmed to believe that disease and health problems are related to genes, yet only 1% of the health problems we face are connected to genes.

There is a health crisis, yet over 90% of health problems are coming from stress. Stress shows itself in various ways depending on which stresses you have. Stress can be caused by anything that gets in the way of where you're going.

Receding Gums

Tooth grinding, lip and tongue piercing, and subtle hormonal changes during puberty, pregnancy, or menopause have also become contributing factors to receding gums, so consider the possibility of one or more of these. Smoking is less of a cause of gum disease, but smoking will exacerbate any deteriorating condition in the mouth.

When gums recede, teeth appear bigger. There is often pain, and the teeth develop sensitivity, often working their way loose and dislodging from the jaw. Because it happens slowly, people with gum disease often do nothing until the condition has set in.

Mouthwash

The Chinese used mouthwash as long ago as 2700 BC. Ayurvedic medicine prescribes mouthwash as a treatment for gum disease. The Romans rinsed their mouths as well as brushing their teeth, using vinegar and Alum (a sulphur-rich salt).

Across the Ionian Sea, the Greeks preferred olive tree leaves, oil, milk, and wine, as well as peelings from pomegranates, gallnuts, and vinegar. North American Indians used mouth rinses derived from plants such as Coptis Trifolia (Threeleaf Goldthread or Savoyane). 18th century Europe found a use for a urine-based mouthwash because of the ammonia content.

If your mouth is in a healthy state, by far the best mouthwash to use is your own saliva. Swallowing it boosts your immune system!

For those of you who are in the habit of using mouthwash every morning or before a date night, I've listed several botanicals and other solutions that'll freshen your mouth better than anything else.

As there are so many ways to create your own mouthwash, you don't need to be restricted to the few I suggest. Try any of these solutions, and you won't need to buy that expensive, chemically-burdened mouthwash ever again. In any case, chemical mouthwashes have been strongly linked to cancers.

I listed certain ingredients in toothpaste to watch out for. Here's the equivalent list for mouthwash:

- Chlorhexidine (can lead to serious heart conditions),
- Alcohol (The Dental Journal of Australia stated alcohol increases the risk of developing oral, head and neck cancers),
- Hexetidine aka Oraldene (may cause clotting in your brain and is considered a carcinogen),
- Methyl Salicylate (beware - a teaspoon of Methyl Salicate is like aspirins on steroids),

- Benzalkonium Chloride (toxic to humans causing skin and mucous membrane irritation when ingested),
- Cetylphyridinium Chloride (causes tooth staining plaque to build up),
- Methparaben (a UK study suggested parabens cause breast cancer) and Corsodyl (see below).

You may think that because you're not swallowing commercial mouthwash, it is safer, but the ingredients come into contact with the sensitive oral mucous membranes where they are absorbed into your body.

Here's an effective mouthwash you can easily make at home:

- 1 tablespoon bicarbonate of soda
- 1/4 teaspoon unrefined salt
- add warm water (to dissolve the salt)
- add stevia to taste

It won't take long to make, after which you can add different ingredients from the list in Part Four.

Whilst on the subject, you may have seen a TV ad where a woman's teeth fall out of her mouth and into her hands. Of course it's a bad dream. Then, as she brushes her teeth, blood comes out of her mouth. Were you shocked? Could blatant scaremongering have been the purpose behind the ad for Corsodyl? The tagline is "Because losing a tooth in real-life is worse than a bad dream."

Corsodyl, a GlaxoSmith Kline product, is supposed to fight gum disease and help numb the pain of mouth ulcers. Unfortunately, it contains chlorhexidine digluconate. The chemical has been linked to serious heart conditions and (after long-term use) the staining of teeth brown. Why didn't they use curcumin instead? In 2011, a verdict of 'death by medical misadventure' was recorded at

Brighton County Court after a patient died from anaphylactic shock after using Corsodyl mouthwash administered to her in a dental practice.

READ THOSE LABELS

In January 2014 the UK's Daily Mail wrote:

> *"Using mouthwash is a 'disaster' for health, increasing the risk of heart attacks and strokes, scientists are warning. Swilling kills off 'good' bacteria that help blood vessels relax – so increasing blood pressure. When healthy volunteers used Corsodyl, a brand containing a powerful antiseptic, their blood pressure rose within hours."*
>
> *Professor Amrita Ahluwalia, who led the study, last night condemned the widespread use of antiseptic mouthwash.*
>
> *She said: "Killing off all these bugs each day is a disaster, when small rises in blood pressure have significant impact on morbidity and mortality from heart disease and stroke."*

Even dentists have voiced their concern as patients are opting to use Corsodyl instead of going to the dentist. The use of Corsodyl only masks the underlying condition. Tsk! Tsk!

Tongue

Few people genuinely clean their tongues when they brush their teeth. As an integral part of the mouth, the tongue needs to be kept as clean as every other part.

Tongue scrapers exist because of the benefits of removing the overnight buildup of bacteria from your tongue. Some people use the inside edge of a spoon to scrape their tongues. That's certainly better than not scraping at all, but if you get yourself a genuine tongue scraper AND USE IT DAILY to scrape oral bacteria away before it builds up, you'll be so much better off.

If you believe your breath stinks, start using a tongue scraper.

Flossing

The most incisive question I've heard in conjunction with flossing was: *"How can you kill an infection with a piece of string?"*

The value of flossing is largely mythical. Flossing does remove large particles of food stuck between your teeth but when it comes to eliminating bacteria from deep under your gums, flossing falls short of the task. To claim that tooth decay is caused because you don't floss enough is, at best, whimsical. There's certainly no research to substantiate this claim.

To compound the issue, sugars and carbohydrates nourish the bacteria in our mouths. An excess of sugar or drinks containing high fructose corn syrup actively multiplies bacteria under your gum line. This should concern you.

In the 1980's, Periodontist Dr Joseph Phillips cautioned us: *"Flossing with string can give you a live bacterial vaccination. Mark my words, a big Class Action suit will be coming against the Dental Society for teaching flossing."*

The Class Action suit didn't occur because the American Dental Association painted Dr. Phillips as a maverick and pressured him into early retirement.

It is vital to keep the balance of bacteria in check to have a healthy mouth. There are some 400-500 different types of bacteria in the mouth, a few of which may be classified as 'rogue' rather than 'bad'.

Flossing may remove food debris, but rather than removing it, flossing tends to spread pathogenic bacteria around your mouth. To have and maintain proper oral (and overall) health, you need to ensure pathogenic bacteria cannot build up in your mouth.

Since floss was first patented in 1874, some dentists have advocated its use. Dental associations have endorsed it, and government bodies have promoted it. Today, some dentists even hand out floss samples to patients to use in their battle against gum disease and tooth decay. *"Floss twice a day"*, they tell patients.

"Except there's little proof that flossing works", writes the Guardian.

> *"Following an investigation by Associated Press (AP), last year (2015) journalists from the agency asked the departments of health and human services and agriculture in the US for their evidence that flossing works.*

> *Since then, the US government has quietly dropped the recommendation, admitting that there is no scientific evidence to prove the benefits. And now the NHS is set to review their own guidelines.*

A leading British dentist said there is only *"weak evidence"* that flossing helps in this way. Professor Damien Walmsley of Birmingham University, said the time and expense required for reliable studies meant the health claims often attributed to floss were unproven.

Walmsley, who is also a scientific adviser to the British Dental Association, said: *"The difficulty is trying to get good evidence. People are different and large studies are costly to do ... until then you can't really say yes or no."* He added *"more sophisticated trials"* were needed. *"It's important to tell people to do the basics. Flossing is not part of the basics."*

AP also looked at the most rigorous research of the past decade. Twenty-five studies in leading journals found evidence for flossing is *"weak, very unreliable"*, of *"very low"* quality, and carries "a moderate to large potential for bias".

One review conducted last year said:

> *"The majority of available studies fail to demonstrate that flossing is generally effective in plaque removal."*

Another 2015 review cites *"inconsistent/weak evidence"* for flossing and a *"lack of efficacy"*. One study did credit floss with a slight reduction in gum inflammation.

A dental magazine commented that any benefit would be so minute that users might not notice.

In my opinion, flossing can cause considerable harm. Poor flossing techniques damage gums by dislodging infection-causing bacteria.

The British Dental Association commented:

> *"Small inter-dental brushes are best for cleaning the area in between the teeth, where there is space to do so. Floss is of little value unless the spaces between your teeth are too tight for the interdental brushes to fit without hurting or causing harm."*

This isn't just me ranting about flossing. Holistic Dentist Dr. Reid L. Winick, D.D.S., says, *"Throw away your floss."*

For those of you who may continue flossing more vigilantly, it's much better for the environment if you use silk floss, which has recently become available at FlossPot.com

For a refreshing perspective on flossing from a dental hygienist.....

Key into YouTube and watch: **Dental Floss Is a Waste Of Time: Today Show** (2:49)

Kissing

When two people kiss and they're both healthy, there's a beneficial exchange of saliva. A 10-second "intimate kiss" can transfer up to 80 million bacteria from mouth to mouth. Both kissers benefit and there's a boost to both immune systems. When kissing involves one or more unhealthy mouths, things don't quite go so well.

Your tongue is generally recognised as the opening to your heart. Your tongue can express emotions such as anger and the hate stored within you as it stimulates passion when used in kissing.

In his book "How To Survive In A World Without Antibiotics" Dr. Keith Scott-Mumby writes:

69

"The mouth is the source of some hideous germs and, in fact, oral sex is far more hygienic than kissing someone! You would worry more about your private parts becoming infected, than the mouth picking up something nasty (let's not be bashful here)."

Oddly enough, he is right. Your mouth is a sex gland that interacts with your genitals, thyroid, and pituitary.

Scott-Mumby continues,

"Remember the words of the Bobby Gentry song:

"What do you get when you kiss a guy? You get enough germs to catch pneumonia..." Medically speaking, she's bang on!"

It gets worse. As Scott-Mumby reveals in the book, if you were to take the open infectious sores around gums and teeth in the average mouth and run them all together, you would have an area of pus equivalent to an open wound covering the back of your hand. Sorry about any mental image that may have created.

Whenever you chew food, the chewing releases showers of bacteria into the blood. The harder you chew, the more bacteria are released. It causes a condition called bacteremia, bacteria floating around free in the blood. Scott-Mumby adds:

"It's been a saying of mine for decades that dentists don't know how many people they kill. There's no feedback; how could they? And doctors don't realise they are looking at a dental work complication, because they don't ask the vital question I just shared. So nobody is joining the dots and getting the full picture. Till now."

Bad Breath

With bad breath, you have to eliminate the cause rather than mask it daily with mouthwash. The build-up of bacteria on the tongue is a major contributor to bad breath. Tongue scraping daily will help with this. If the condition persists, your intestines may become sluggish. An indicator of this is smelly armpits. If your breath continues to smell after that, you need to book a deep colon cleanse.

In the meantime, take some probiotics daily - foods such as kimchi and sauerkraut, pineapple and mango and drink pure water. The bacteria in fermented foods help suppress the growth of plaque and gingivitis, causing pathogens in the mouth.

Although unlikely, you may have tonsil stones. Ask your Dental Hygienist to determine whether this is the case.

Lemon juice diluted with some water will go a long way to destroying bad breath but remember not to use it more than once a week as the acidity of lemon juice can damage tooth enamel.

Part Four:

Effective Natural Remedies

The next few pages contain lists of botanicals and other well-established remedies you can use instead of commercial toothpastes and mouthwashes. Become familiar with them. If you've not used any of them before, start with sensible amounts in case of allergic reactions or dosage misunderstandings. Recommended doses will be on the labels.

If you really have to take capsules so be it. Personally I prefer direct contact with the substances themselves.

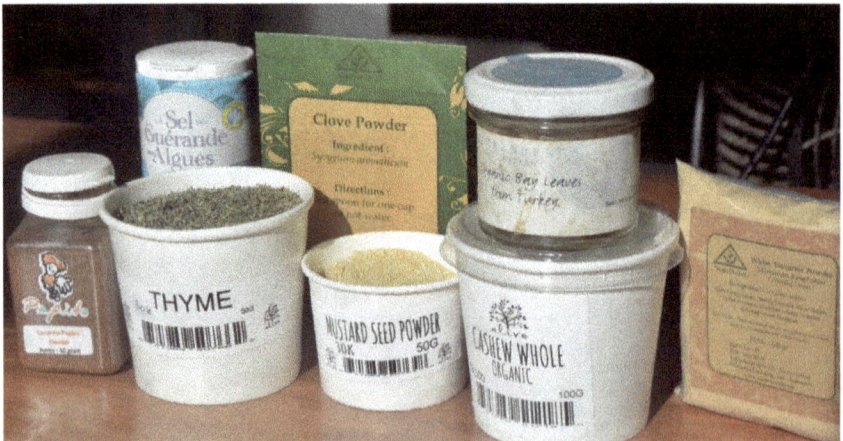

Part of my 'stash', from Left to Right: Cayenne Pepper, Thyme, Celtic Sea Salt, Clove Powder, Mustard Seed

Powder, Cashews, Bay Leaves and White Turmeric Powder

I'll give brief details on each in alphabetical order. The list is sufficient rather than exhaustive. I've often come across questionable internet opinions on essential oils and how they can damage the microbiology in the mouth.

Whether essential oils are "harmful" or "not harmful" depends on the circumstances. By nature, essences from plants are strong medicine and should not be taken undiluted as damage to sensitive gum tissue could occur.

Even diluted essential oils can cause burning and irritation to sensitive mucous membranes. I occasionally rinse with a few drops of neem oil in water. How much water? For me, this is determined by the taste of the result. For me, that's about half a small glass. How often do I do this? Once or twice a month at most. I came to this conclusion after consulting a certified aromatherapist.

If you're on any medication or suffer from allergies, make sure you speak with your practitioner before trying out something you're not already familiar with. Some natural substances may have side effects if taken in combination with certain drugs.

Activated Charcoal is an effective antidote for detoxing heavy metals and halting the impact of many poisons. For this reason, It is used in many Emergency Units and paramedic ambulances and is a popular ingredient in homemade toothpaste. It binds with toxins as it passes through the gastrointestinal tract, even in the mouth if you have amalgam fillings. Dentists should let their patients rinse with it before removing amalgam fillings and rinse the cavities afterwards. Activated charcoal is also reputed to prevent toxins from making their way to your heart. It is best used at a different time from any medicines you may take in case the benefits of the medicine are removed before they have time to take effect.

Occasionally, I've read of dentists' unsubstantiated concerns that activated charcoal is abrasive to enamel. Truthfully, that's just professional scaremongering. I've never found anything to substantiate that; indeed, it is well-known for its ability to remove stains from enamel. I add water to Activated Charcoal and rinse it around my mouth before brushing it onto and around my teeth as I spit it out. Ensure it is food-grade activated charcoal and that it is sourced from wood or coconut rather than petroleum-based.

Key into YouTube and watch: **How Charcoal Can Change Your Life** (2:03)

Aloe Vera is a truly remarkable remedy for bleeding or swollen gums. Cut an aloe leaf and squeeze the mineral and vitamin-rich gel onto a clean fingertip or clean cloth, gently rubbing it onto the infected area. Aloe vera is popular as an anti-fungal and anti-inflammatory wound healer that helps combat candida, Streptococcus Mutans, gingivitis, and periodontitis.

Aloe vera can be used as a tooth gel (especially for those with sensitive teeth) and is a good alternative to fluoride without the potential side effects. If you have ill-fitting dentures, the use of aloe vera will offset any bacterial contamination and inflammatory irritations. Commercial aloe products are available, but the plant is so easy to grow even indoors, so what's stopping you?

Apple Cider Vinegar is full of beneficial enzymes, pectin and trace minerals. It has a strong taste and pH similar to battery acid. It must be used with a great deal of common sense caution as it can wear down the protective enamel of your teeth. Used primarily against bad breath, chronic gum infections, oral thrush and tooth stains, Apple Cider Vinegar, with a sprinkling of bicarbonate of soda generously diluted with water, can be a practical ingredient for any homemade mouthwash.

Basil leaves To freshen and disinfect the mouth, chew two or three of these every day. Basil has astringent properties that help 'tighten' the gums and destroy the bacteria responsible for plaque and bad breath. Either chew the leaves, add them to water, and use them as a mouth rinse, or chop the leaves into tiny pieces and include them in your homemade toothpaste.

Bay Leaf, nicknamed "Jewish Penicillin," has been used for hundreds of years in minor surgeries for its bacteria-killing properties, specifically members of the streptococcus family, mould, fungus, and the harmful yeast candida albicans. Shred the leaves and mix them with water to include them in any homemade toothpaste, as they have tooth-whitening properties.

Bentonite Clay is a healing clay, especially rich in magnesium, calcium and silica. Because of its ability to absorb toxins and soak up heavy metals and other impurities, it helps cleanse and heal the body internally and externally. Resulting from the weathering of volcanic ash in the presence of water, clay is alkaline and has been used as a means of warding off disease for centuries by tribal cultures in Africa, Australia and South America.

Safe for children and to consume internally, I recommend you take small amounts to begin with, as too much may swell within your body, causing mild discomfort from temporary intestinal blockages. The mouth is one of the most susceptible areas of the body when it comes to harmful outside invaders taking over. Bentonite Clay is a useful ingredient in homemade toothpaste.

There are many ways to take it. I sprinkle it over my muesli at breakfast.

Bicarbonate of Soda (aka baking soda) has been used to clean teeth for well over 150 years and remains a popular ingredient in homemade toothpaste and mouthwashes. Indeed it may be the simplest and least expensive preventative available as it:

- raises alkalinity in the mouth neutralising the harmful effects of bacterial acids.
- strengthens the enamel by helping to increase calcium absorption
- "buffers" off plaque on the teeth enamel without damaging the enamel

Despite attempts to smear bicarbonate of soda as an enamel stripper, it is very gentle on the enamel as a polishing agent.

I can personally attest to the effectiveness of brushing with a mixture of bicarbonate of soda and coconut oil once a week, sometimes replacing coconut oil with lemon juice. Bicarbonate of soda can remove stains, absorb smells (improving the quality of breath), whiten teeth, and kill harmful bacteria.

Cacao is the most natural form of chocolate. The cacao plant contains heart-healthy polyphenols, which lower blood pressure and reduce 'bad' cholesterol. They also contribute more effectively to the remineralisation of tooth enamel than fluoride.

Calendula Tea is one of those "all-rounders" that range from helping restore poor skin conditions to alleviating haemorrhoids, menstrual pain and stomach ulcers. Often mistaken for marigolds, calendula is so much more than an ornamental plant. It can be used in mouthwashes and mixed into toothpaste (highly recommended). It also contributes to reducing gum swellings, cavitation, plaque and gingivitis.

Cardamom is indisputably one of the healthiest herbs on our planet. For centuries, Cardamom has been a popular remedy in Ayurvedic and Traditional Chinese Medicine. Referred to as the "Queen of Spices", the pods are commonly chewed in India to freshen breath, stimulate saliva flow and prevent cavity development. One ingredient, cineole, is a powerful antiseptic that targets the bacteria causing bad breath. For this reason alone, cardamom is often used to flavour chewing gums. Rich in phytonutrients, manganese (good for bones), and Vitamin C, cardamom helps stop bleeding gums.

Cayenne Pepper has been used for thousands of years to treat digestive issues, heart problems, chronic pain, poor circulation, sore throats, headaches, toothache and increased brain function. The principal medicinal properties come from capsaicin; flavonoids in cayenne pepper are known to repair heart cells. The vitamins A, C, B6 and K destroy bacteria.

Treat cayenne pepper with caution if you're not good at handling spicy foods.

No other herb increases your blood flow faster than cayenne pepper. This is important for teeth, gums and the jaw bone. When part of your body is sick, there is often a blood restriction within that area. Blood flow is vital because it carries nutrition and oxygen to that area and removes waste debris. Cayenne pepper acts like a controlled implosion, blasting through the blockages to reach the sick area, taking with it all the minerals and vitamins from the foods you eat and all the vital chemicals from the herbs you take.

Peppers are measured by their heat units, determining their usage and value. The rule of thumb is the hotter the pepper, the more capsaicin it contains. These are great if you find cayenne pepper labelled 40,000, 60,000, 90,000 or more heat units. The lower-heat cayenne pepper, around 30,000 heat units, is much less efficient and generally contaminated. These are the ones to avoid.

If you're not used to cayenne pepper, work your way up. Mix it with a pinch of water or juice; stir and drink. Get to know it and how your body responds to it. Then increase your dose. The real value of cayenne pepper is not staying at these lower doses. Ultimately you want to get to a level where your ears pop, your toes curl upward, and you think, *"Holy Moses!"* every time you take it. That's when it's doing you some real good.

Much of cayenne pepper's healing action takes place in your mouth. As it touches your tongue, it is absorbed in seconds, and nerve endings produce signals that send waves of fresh blood throughout your body. This is a handy resource to have if someone in your home has a heart attack.

CBD (Cannabidiol) minimises the risk of gum disease and can counteract the underlying inflammation that leads to conditions such as periodontitis. Periodontitis causes gums to pull away from the teeth, making them more likely to become infected. This can break down the bones and tissues supporting teeth, resulting in tooth loss.

CBD oil can also help with inflammation, pain, neurological issues, and more. Unlike THC s non-psychoactive, which means it doesn't cause a "high".

Try using CBD oil if you have:

- Any anxiety or dental phobia
- Chronic dental/oral pain
- Sensitivity to hot and cold
- Receding gums
- Gum disease (periodontitis, gingivitis, etc.)

Chia Seeds (see Sesame Seeds)

Cinnamon is impressive at keeping bacteria at bay, particularly Streptococcus Mutans. Apart from being great with food (especially for those with diabetes), you can rinse your mouth with cinnamon powder and water or add it to a glass of bicarbonate of soda, pure water, lemon juice, or apple cider vinegar. I regularly add cinnamon to my coffee; every time I open a mango or melon, I sprinkle cinnamon on the flesh before eating. Cinnamon is definitely one for the dental first aid kit.

Cloves are the best-known of all toothache remedies. It has remarkable anti-inflammatory and disinfectant properties that help reduce harmful 'bad bugs' that cause gum swellings. Whenever I had mouth ulcers, I regularly took a whole clove and popped it into my mouth close to the ulcer. After a short while, I'd feel a numbing effect. This approach is infinitely better for dealing with bad breath than any commercial mouthwash I know of. I'll add the precaution here: if you're on any medication for blood clotting, speak with your doctor first.

Coconut Oil The Athlone Institute of Technology in Ireland suggested that people use coconut oil treated with enzymes to manage levels of bacteria, particularly the harmful bacteria Streptococcus Mutans. Coconut oil is a wonderful base for homemade mouthwashes and toothpastes. Dr Bruce Fife ND points out that the value of coconut oil crossing the brain barrier is to have a product high in lauric acid bathing our brains and bodies daily. This is particularly beneficial against the onset of brain and neurodegenerative disorders. Different bacteria and viruses believed to reside in our mouths have been found in the brains of Alzheimer's patients.

Colloidal Silver Reputed to be able to destroy 650 different bacteria, fungi and viruses in 72 Hours, colloidal silver is beneficial. So why have the health authorities of many countries banned it? If you're living in one of the 'banned' countries, you can instead buy a colloidal silver maker and produce it yourself. That's what I do. As for its application, I usually rinse my mouth with it (undiluted) and include it as an ingredient in my homemade toothpaste. The germicidal properties of silver were recognised as early as 70 B.C. Before the advent of refrigerators, your grandparents would put silver coins in their milk to prolong its freshness.

In the early 1900s, scientists discovered that the body's most essential fluids were colloidal: blood transports nutrition and oxygen to the cells. In the presence of pathogens (viruses, bacteria or fungi), colloidal silver disables their oxygen enzyme, causing the pathogen to suffocate and die. The pathogen is then expelled from the body. This process does not harm the beneficial enzymes or the human body's chemistry. The result is the destruction of disease-causing organisms in the body and the food. Where pharmaceutical antibiotics destroy beneficial enzymes, colloidal silver leaves beneficial enzymes intact. Thus, colloidal silver is absolutely safe for humans, reptiles, plants and all multi-celled living matter.

Dill Seeds and Leaves are extremely good breath fresheners. They help reduce damage caused to teeth and gums by free radicals. Crush the seeds or cut the leaves into small pieces and add them to homemade mouthwash and toothpaste.

Eucalyptus leaves As with many botanicals, the value of eucalyptus is its bacteria-killing and inflammation-relieving properties. If you try a eucalyptus mouthwash, diluting it with water will offset any strong taste until you become used to it. Because of its anti-microbial properties, Eucalyptus oil is an ingredient in several mouthwash and dental preparations, as the oil may possess anti-microbial properties.

Garlic is a painkiller and helps remedy gum disease. Rub a broken clove of raw garlic around the painful area of your gums. If you add to toothpaste or mouthwash, keep the amounts low to avoid 'garlic breath'.

Ginger contains the active ingredient raffinose, known to reduce the build-up of bacteria-induced biofilm on teeth. I use ginger in my morning juices and add slices when cooking fish suppers. If you have a toothache, bite into a slice of ginger for fast relief. Ginger and lemon tea is high on my list of favourites.

Ginkgo Biloba is another reliable ancient remedy, known for improving blood flow in and around the diseased gum or tooth. This results in the regeneration of gum tissue and tooth bone.

Ginseng (Asian): While neither a gum healer nor a pain reducer for toothache, it would be remiss of me not to include ginseng in a list of beneficial botanicals if only for its benefits within periodontal tissues (cementum, the periodontal ligament, alveolar bone, and gingival tissue). Be careful not to overuse it. In case of allergies, try small amounts first.

Grapeseed Extract, available in liquid or powder form, is effective at remineralising teeth. A natural compound found in grapeseed extract is believed to strengthen dentin. Researchers at the Chicago College of Dentistry believe that grapeseed extract can extend the life of your teeth.

Green Tea A cup of green tea daily has been shown to reduce gum pocket depth, reduce bleeding, and help minimise gum tissue loss. The natural phenol in green tea helps to destroy periodontal disease and reduce inflammation, strengthening the connection between the gums and teeth. In one study at the University of Texas, green tea extract was given to patients with precancerous lesions in their mouths, and it slowed the progression to oral cancer. Animal studies have also found that tea compounds can inhibit cancer growth.

Guava Leaves are rich in flavonoids and have been used for centuries throughout India and the Middle East to reduce gum disease (especially bleeding gums) and the pain of loosening teeth. Chewing a guava leaf twice a day is recommended to achieve this, and results have been been seen within a few days of starting.

Hemp Oil/Hemp Seed Oil Hemp oil helps with bad breath and any sensitivity in your teeth and gums. An alternative to coconut oil for oil pulling, this process can strengthen your teeth, heal bleeding gums, and prevent gingivitis and bad breath. I often add a teaspoon of hemp seed oil to my morning juices.

Honey (Manuka): the inherent peroxide in honey makes it one of the best antibacterial and antiviral products. Honey can heal wounds inside and outside the mouth and act as a barrier to infection, keeping wounds moist while healing. As early as 1200, there are records of honey being used for healing. Today, the use of honey as a salve helps heal mouth ulcers or minor gum and tongue sores. It is, of course, a valuable cough remedy.

Hydrogen Peroxide (H2O2): If you can source it, you ideally want 35% Food-Grade. Applied too often or for too long, it'll damage tooth enamel. The H2O2 found in dental cleaning kits is at such low dosages it's almost ineffective. If you can't get it in your country, use Manuka Honey instead, as it contains higher levels of enzymes that create natural hydrogen peroxide.

Note: 3% H2O2 that has already been diluted and classified as food-grade is available in most countries, but it's not the real deal. Otherwise, in the UK, 35% Food Grade H2O2 is only sold directly to licensed businesses with certificates.

Iodine: I cannot say enough about iodine. It's an essential micronutrient and must be in every 21st-century First Aid Kit. A few drops of iodine in a small glass of water is all you need. Rinse around your mouth for a few minutes to eliminate bad bugs. Some people are allergic to iodine, so if you're unsure, first test it on your skin.

Key into YouTube and watch:

- **Fluoride Does Not Reduce Tooth Decay-But THIS Does! (6:57)** Brilliant Info!
- **Iodine - Suppressed knowledge that can change your life**

Kratom has been used for hundreds of years by Southeast Asian cultures as a powerful anti-oxidant that, amongst its extensive range of benefits, has been found to reduce neuron damage following a stroke. There are different strains available, red vein kratom being the most popular for its pain-killing effects (toothache).

Again, it's popular, and Kratom is going through a backlash from the scientific press as I write. It's claimed that too much Kratom can be harmful. I respectfully suggest that too much of anything can be harmful so that the argument doesn't pass the rationale test.

Like everything, use common sense and read the dosage guide on the label.

Lemon juice is acidic externally and becomes alkaline once swallowed. Here, we're using it to rinse the mouth. Excessive use can damage the enamel, but the many properties are wonderful for stimulating the re-growth of receding gums. Once a week, I squeeze the juice from half a lemon and mix it with a pinch of bicarbonate of soda before rinsing it around my mouth for a minute or so. After spitting it out, I brush my teeth with a bamboo toothbrush. Only then does my entire mouth feel clean.

Moringa is one of those outstanding plants. Gram for gram contains four times the calcium of eight ounces of milk, twice the protein, four times the vitamin A of carrots, three times the iron of spinach, three times the potassium of bananas, and the vitamin C equivalent of seven oranges. Highly beneficial to human health, moringa is a valuable, calcium-rich weapon against bone and tooth loss.

Whatever your health condition, take moringa regularly. It is also valuable for preventing muscle contraction, problems associated with central nervous function, and hormone secretion. The leaves contain an abundance of zeatin, which is believed to delay cell ageing. Ayurvedic medicine currently uses moringa as a natural restorative for over 300 diseases.

Mustard Oil is rich in vitamins and has valuable antioxidant properties. Place half a teaspoon of mustard oil in the palm of your hand, and with a clean finger or cloth, rub the oil gently into the gums. Rinse with water when finished. Mustard oil stimulates the gums, increases blood circulation, and soothes any pain. It can be used daily.

Myrrh is an old-timer in Egyptian, Chinese, Arab and African cultures. Known to stop deterioration in gum conditions, using myrrh gum powder in homemade toothpaste helps keep the mouth healthy. Mix it into a paste by adding a little water. Massage the mix into your gums with a clean finger or cloth.

Nutmeg & Mace: With antibacterial properties, nutmeg and mace have long been used in cooking and for medical benefits. The oils of both have been used to relieve bad breath, toothaches, mouth sores, and that old favourite, flatulence.

Neem is a living pharmacy, a great destroyer of rogue bacteria. I first encountered it in the 1960s when the cargo ship I was on was unloading freight in Aden. As I walked around the docks, one of the lasting impressions I had was of men sitting in a cafe with small sticks protruding from their mouths. I was told this was their way of cleaning their teeth.

The neem sticks, which have frayed ends, are made from either the neem or mustard seed tree and are used to remove food particles from between teeth. In the West, people spend 45 seconds cleaning their teeth in the morning; the Arabs I watched spent over 30 minutes with the neem stick in their mouths.

Oregano powder is a powerful broad-spectrum application that is bactericidal and fungicidal with no side effects. Unlike antibiotics, there have been no instances of bacterial resistance. The active ingredient, carvacrol, is why oregano is already in your kitchen; it breaks through the outer wall of norovirus species - those that cause food-borne illnesses. Given its strong antibacterial and antibiotic properties, rub pure, undiluted oregano oil around an infected tooth or place a drop or two of it on your bristles when brushing. Even with small doses, plaque does not build up on your teeth, and the health of your gums will improve dramatically.

Parsley

Besides its well-known enzyme-deodorising ability to freshen breath quickly (even garlic breath), the vitamin C content and volatile oil compounds help strengthen loose teeth. Note that parsley relieves a condition rather than curing it. Include parsley in your diet more often to benefit from the many other properties, including repairing damaged tissues, managing blood pressure, eliminating moulds from your body and processing oxygen.

Peppermint: If you're worried about your breath, carry around a small spray bottle of food-grade peppermint oil. A single spray into our mouth is so much more effective than chewing gum and without the side effects. To help with bad breath, add peppermint leaves to hot water and allow them to steep for 20-30 minutes. Rinse your mouth thoroughly and spit out.

Propolis, or "bee glue," supplies a broad spectrum of vitamins, minerals, and trace elements, which are vital to the overall health of the mouth.

Quinton Marine Plasma represents the original blueprint of life and contains three times the mineral concentration of your blood. If you need rapid mineralisation, this is what you need to take. In a rather unusual experiment, the developer, Rene Quinton, confirmed his hypothesis by draining a dog of all its blood to the point of no reflex from even its eyelids. He then replaced the removed blood volume with Marine Plasma. Not only did the dog survive, but having recovered, the dog became more active and healthy than before.

Positive Health magazine reported:

> *"Quinton's first human treatment was in a Parisian hospital for a comatose man expected to die the same day from Typhoid. Within just a few hours of the first intravenous dose of QMP, the man emerged from his coma, started eating and talking and went on to make a full recovery following further treatment. Quinton had a similar result with a man with cirrhosis of the liver and erysipelas."*

Healthy blood travelling throughout all parts of the body is imperative. QMP is definitely one of my go-to products when I'm feeling run down.

Rosemary Crush fresh leaves to massage the gums with rosemary oil. This will boost circulation and help the healing process. Steep some rosemary leaves in a glass of warm to hot water before swishing around your mouth. This not only help to eliminate bacteria but also improves your breath.

Sage has valuable cleansing properties and has been a popular home remedy for centuries. To try it for yourself, either use dried sage or chop up a fresh sage leaf and pack it onto the swollen gum area for a few minutes.

Salt Water Rinse Add a heaped teaspoonful of mineral-rich, unrefined sea salt to warm water and rinse it around your mouth. This basic solution works sufficiently well although some people 'upgrade' it by adding bicarbonate of soda or herbal tinctures.

Sesame Seeds (small seeds in general) are great at removing plaque. Ask your favourite anthropologist about the condition of the teeth in those skeletons they are forever digging up. Sesame seeds are high in calcium (the building block of your teeth) and help preserve tooth and jaw bone quality.

Sweet Wormwood (Artemisia annua) has been a popular botanical, especially for its antibacterial and antifungal properties. I once asked a Master Herbalist from Damascus why he hadn't used this ingredient in his anti-parasite remedies. He answered that taken repeatedly over a period of months, wormwood has the potential to become addictive. The story goes that when painter Van Gogh cut off his ear, he was under the influence of the wormwood-based drink Absinthe.

Tea Tree Oil is an exceptionally potent antiseptic and a fast-acting ingredient in any mouthwash. I have written that I prefer not to take essential oils orally, but clove, tea tree, and peppermint oils are common in mouthwash recipes. Use with caution. Some genuine toothpastes include tea tree oil, but again, READ THE LABELS to check out the other ingredients before you buy. A study at Switzerland's Institute of Preventive Dentistry and Oral Microbiology in Basel concluded that tea tree oil decreases the bacterial colonies that cause halitosis, making it beneficial for oral health.

Thieves Oil: A blend of anti-infectious essential oils: clove, lemon, cinnamon, eucalyptus, and rosemary. You can diffuse it to kill mould and bacteria, take it internally to boost immune health, use it topically and enhance the health of teeth and gums for toothache or inflammation.

Turmeric has become one of the most commonly promoted botanicals on social media platforms, primarily due to its power in reducing inflammation. A 2012 issue of the Journal of Indian Society of Periodontology credited turmeric mouthwash with being effective in controlling plaque and preventing gingivitis.

Turmeric Removes Fluoride From The Brain

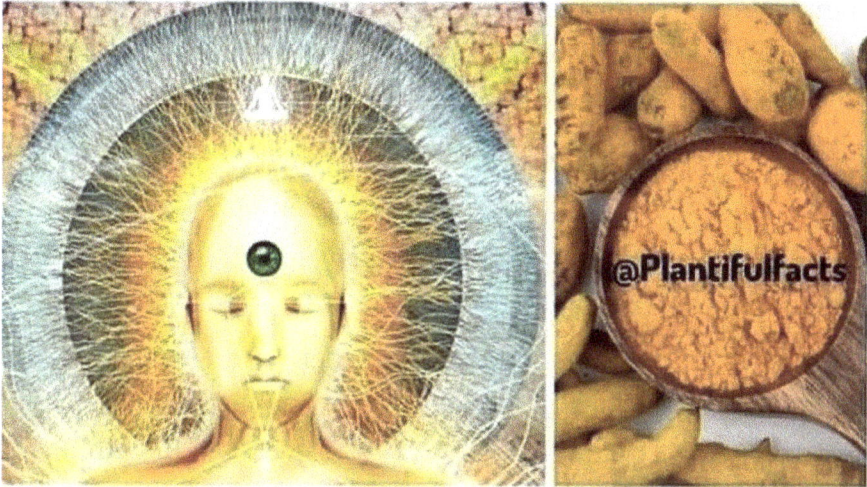

Curcumin, found in turmeric, appears to raise endogenous glutathione production in the brain, a major antioxidant defense system. The study investigated the mechanisms through which fluoride induces severe neurodegenerative changes in the mammalian brain, particularly in cells of the hippocampus and cerebral cortex

A herbal/medical crossover, turmeric's key ingredient is curcumin, a yellow-pigmented polyphenol revealed as a natural alternative to the often recommended mouthwash ingredient chlorhexidine for gum tissue inflammation. According to news-medical.net, *"Curcurmin can improve and boost levels of the brain hormone brain-derived neurotrophic factor (BDNF), which promotes the growth of new neurons and wards off many degenerative processes in the brain. Hence, turmeric has been used to attempt to prevent diseases such as Alzheimer's disease."* The value placed on turmeric is such that Indian brides use its distinguishing hue on their wedding day.

My personal preference is to drink turmeric in the traditional Javanese beverage, 'Jamu', adding a sprinkling of ground pepper to help the beneficial ingredients cross the blood-brain barrier. Occasionally, I mix a teaspoon of turmeric powder with some Manuka honey to form a paste, leaving it in my mouth for several minutes so it coats my teeth and gums. When finished, I swallow it before rinsing my mouth with water.

If you are on medication to reduce stomach acid, turmeric should not be used as the body will increase its production of stomach acid. This may induce bloating, nausea, stomach pains and damage to the oesophagus.

There was an attempt to patent turmeric's active ingredient, curcumin, for its health benefits. Ever since the U.S. Patent Office rejected the application, certain elements within the pharmaceutical industry have been discrediting turmeric as best they can.

Unrefined Sea Salt has proven useful in helping to remedy infected gums. When you next go swimming at the beach, rinse your mouth out repeatedly with seawater. Check first for nearby sewage outlets just in case! I used to rinse this way as a teenager when I had mouth ulcers. This simple approach was very healing. If you live far from the sea, buy some unrefined sea salt, add a healthy pinch of it to pure water and swish it around your mouth for a couple of minutes before spitting it out. The salt dries out the membrane within the gums as the water helps flush out rogue bacteria.

Urine You read that right. It may sound disgusting but urine was used by the Romans to whiten their teeth. Made up of 95% water, urine contains over 3000 compounds including ammonia. That's what removes stains. Many people have told me that the healthier the food you eat, the better the taste of urine. If you're game to try it I'd suggest diluting it to begin with, reducing the dilution as you become braver!

Vitamin C Never lose sight of this amazing substance, especially for gum health. Intravenous Vitamin C is the best you can get but some practitioners make unsubstantiated claims as to what it can achieve. While small amounts of Vitamin C can prevent conditions such as scurvy, larger doses are not harmful - indeed they can save lives. Be careful when buying Vitamin C as the often discounted store-bought pills are predominantly made from calcium carbonate (chalk). Bleeding gums often indicate a Vitamin C deficiency. To boost your vitamin C levels, eat more vegetables and fruits (organic if you can), especially garlic.

Although not necessarily a remedy for teeth and gums, probiotics can work wonders for the bacterial balance of your mouth. Once again I mention *Streptococcus Mutans,* a significant contributor to bad breath. Supplementing with probiotics helps keep your gut as well as your mouth healthy. If you genuinely need some extra help, oral probiotic rinses are available too.

Probiotics such as Acidophilus and Bifidus create a healthy biofilm that surrounds the tooth, protecting it. When that biofilm breaks down you can become addicted to the substances that caused the breakdown, usually antibiotics. What commonly causes your biofilm to break down? Commercial mouthwash and synthetic toothpaste.

[Note: I'm obliged to write that no governmental body regulates herbs and supplements. There is thus no guarantee of strength, purity or safety of products; effects may vary. Always read product labels. If you have a medical condition or are taking other drugs,

herbs, or supplements, you should speak with a qualified healthcare provider before embarking on any new regimen. Consult your healthcare provider immediately if you experience side effects.]

Toothbrushing in Japan

It has long been recognised that the Japanese are amongst the healthiest and longest-living nations in the world. In 2008 Japan had more than 33,000 people older than 100 years. On 17 September 2016, this figure had risen to 67,824.

The Japanese are renowned for their ability to turn something that may appear ordinary to us in the Westwern world into something uniquely impressive. We've all been amazed to witness their techniques of folding paper, Origami (or Kirigami if the paper is cut). Yet there are many other Japanese skills we are less aware of.

When Japanese art exploded onto the world stage in the 1860s, it changed everything and was an inspiration for the Impressionist movement in Europe and America. The west then discovered the unique styles of Japanese architecture and religious sculptures as well as Shodo (painting with a small brush), Ukiyo-e (woodblock printing), Manga (the dark comic strips), Bonseki (miniature landscape gardens of sand and stones), Sensu (folding fans used in rituals and dances), Maki-e (luxury lacquerware decorated with gold or silver), Amigurumi, (knitting or crocheting small stuffed animals), Chochin, (collapsible bamboo lanterns), Temari, (embroidered silk balls), Irezumi, (rich tattoos originally to mark criminals), Byobu (folding screens), Gyotaku (printed images of fish caught by fishermen), Samurai Masks (designed to protect the face and strike fear into the heart of an opponent),

Netsuke (hand-crafted sculptures) and of course their martial art Karate (meaning "empty hand").

For those of you who think I missed Bonsai from the list, Bonsai originated in China. Although the word 'Bon-sai' is Japanese, the art of growing dwarf trees in small containers had originated in China by 700 AD.

Back to dental health....Hamigaki is the Japanese art of toothbrushing. In Japan, teeth-related products are a much bigger deal than in many other places. Japanese advertising campaigns in this field are immense.

The Japanese consider tooth brushing as a family bonding activity. Such is the importance attributed to this undertaking that it is also done as a group activity in the classroom every day. Over the years, several tooth-brushing songs focusing on the fun sound effects of hamigaki has been created to keep kids' attention.

Impressively, Japanese statistics reveal that some 50% of adults brush their teeth after every meal, even if that means brushing in the office or in public.

Often brushing is carried out without toothpaste, using just water.

It's also worth noting that few of the Japanese toothpaste brands contain fluoride. Japanese research published in 2010 reported that men and women who drink one or more cups of green tea a day were more likely to hold on to their natural teeth.

Timing and an empty stomach are the most important part of the ancient therapy. It is also recommended to drink warm water during and immediately after meals, wait for 2 hours between meals and drink more warm water.

Teeth Clicking

The old saying goes: "Click your teeth together thirty-six times in the early morning, and your teeth won't fall out when you are old."

You can do this as you wake up or in front of the bathroom mirror, as it only takes 90 seconds at most. Be sure to click your teeth together lightly during this exercise.

First, tap the molars together, then the front teeth, then the canines. Each time, click them 36 times. Saliva will be secreted. Before swallowing, move the saliva around your teeth and gums.

Meridians

"Each tooth is related to an acupuncture meridian which is related to various organs, tissues and glands in the body on this particular meridian or 'energy highway'. This connection is so apparent that an experienced dentist can often assess your overall health and wellness by reviewing your dental condition. If a person has a weak internal organ the condition of the associated meridian tooth could make it considerably more problematic."
American Bio-Compatible Health Systems Inc.

Useo your browser to see the amazing **Tooth Charts** (English, French, Portuguese, Spanish and Chinese versions) on www.dr-elmar-jung.com

Tibetan Water Method

As a nation, Tibetans have enjoyed the benefits of water therapy dating back to ancient times. It is very simple to carry out: drink four glasses of warm water upon waking up. For the next 45 minutes, eat or drink nothing else.

There aren't many dentists in mountainous Tibet, so the monks developed their own way of keeping their teeth and gums healthy. First, they boil water and let it cool down. Then, pouring half a glass of cooled water into the glass, they add one level tablespoon of iodine-free salt, stirring it well. Any residue from the surface is removed.

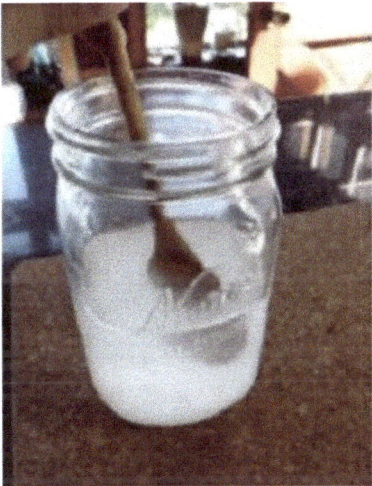

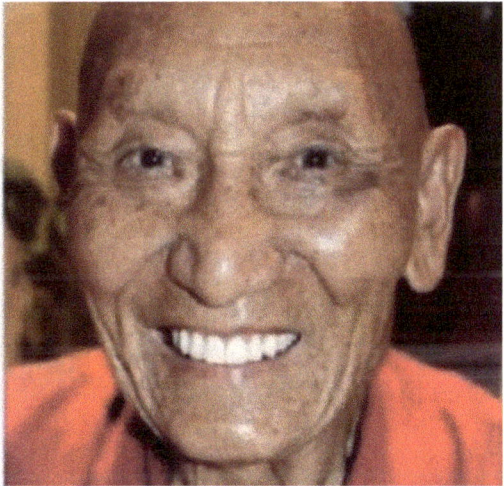

When it settles, salt crystals are visible in the water. Place some crystals on the bristles of your toothbrush and begin cleaning your teeth as you would normally.

The 'salt crystal' toothpaste kills oral pathogens and helps cement any cracks on your tooth enamel.

The Taoist Perspective on Chewing and Saliva

I'll state it here again. Your own saliva is the best mouthwash available, but only when you are healthy. It provides essential minerals to strengthen the tiny cells in your teeth. I'll expand on that here, as the Taoist approach is particularly enlightening. Some facts first (some reiterated for emphasis).

We create between 2 and 4 pints (1 to 2 litres) of saliva every day. Saliva is a fluid containing 99.5% water. The rest is made up of electrolytes, mucus, antibacterial compounds, enzymes, and a painkiller six times more powerful than morphine called Opiorphin - and without the side effects of morphine! Drinking water boosts your saliva levels, which in turn helps resist any buildup of plaque

TaoOfMedicine.com is a helpful website. It explains the makeup of saliva from the perspective of Traditional Chinese Medicine. Saliva consists of *xian* and *tuo*, two different fluids from different origins. *Xian* relates to the earth, that is to say, spleen *qi* and *Tuo* to the water, kidney *qi*. In particular, without *Xian*, you'll have some problem tasting food.

Western medicine acknowledges the importance of saliva to the taste buds. Many patients with chronic or acute pain conditions, sleep disorders, or stress have dry mouths or even dry lips. In such conditions, acupuncture helps to fill their mouths with saliva, often quickly.

They add:

- to prevent overeating, chew until the food turns to liquid in the mouth

- chewing properly lubricates and protects the oesophagus
- once in the stomach, well-chewed food is more easily coated with digestive juices
- less energy is used to digest well-chewed food than hastily chewed/swallowed food.
- saliva moistens the molecules of dry foods to improve their taste
- chewing well allows the nutrients from food to be more quickly absorbed
- chewing for longer allows the flavours to be recognised by the tongue

When healthy, your saliva acts as a first defence against bacterial infection.

If you cut yourself and there's nothing around to use to stem the bleeding, spread your saliva over the wound. This approach will clean the injury and help destroy germs that may cause a subsequent infection. By chewing food well and creating more surface area on which the saliva can act, more potential food-borne bacteria can be killed.

Produced by the parotid glands, saliva is a serous solution containing amylase, a digestive enzyme. The glands are located internally below the ears; the outlet ducts are close to your upper row of molar (back) teeth. The function of saliva is to help with chewing, swallowing and pre-digesting food, as an antibacterial and purifier and to help prevent tooth decay.

Your saliva contains minerals to support the tooth-remineralisation process; the cells in your teeth using these minerals to strengthen themselves. What's important is that saliva maintains the pH of your mouth.

Earlier, I suggested you consider chewing your food more. This creates more saliva, which is used to digest food. These days, people tend to eat their food quickly and move on to the next thing, often a TV programme. Bar the occasional Sunday roast with the family, meals are no longer a family event to enjoy, with food as important as family conversations.

Our ancestors would eat together. Two major contributors to traditional family life has been broken up by central heating and TV.

The slowing down process has two benefits. It allows saliva to build up as a preparation for digesting the food and slows down the rate at which food is digested. Over time, accelerated digestion (and thus, a lack of saliva) has caused several health issues.

If you respect the power of healing water, you'll understand why Taoism considers saliva to be sacred *"...the spiritual fluid of the body"* or *"Heavenly Water."*

Saliva Stimulation Exercise: Saliva will be secreted as you roll your tongue around your mouth and across your teeth. Allow it to collect before swishing it around your mouth for a minute or more before swallowing.

The Patakara Lip Trainer is an exceptional Japanese design that helps restore a wide range of poor health conditions, from snoring and increasing saliva flow to reducing gum inflammation and bad breath.

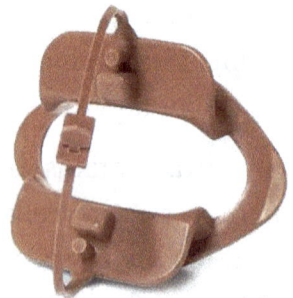

The really important question to ask yourself is, *"Am I a nose or mouth*

breather?" If you don't know, ask your partner to watch you when you sleep.

There's a world of difference between the two. In simple terms breathing through the nose offers many health benefits; breathing through the mouth is shallow. The resultant diminished exchange of gases reduces our cellular energy, depriving us of many health-giving actions that nose breathing provides for our inner organs. Chronic mouth breathing can cause the muscles that open the sidewalls of the nose to weaken through lack of use.....and mouth breathing is known to result in considerably more cavities.

Let's not forget that old phrase, *"Use it or lose it!"*

Whatever makes it difficult for you to breathe through your nose contributes to your breathing through the mouth. Mouth breathing elevates your blood pressure and heart rate, depriving your heart, brain, and other organs of proper oxygenation while exacerbating asthma, sleep apnea, allergies, and rhinitis.

Several studies over the years have evidenced that strengthening the muscles in the oral airway, including the lips, will promote improvement of tongue position and may reduce the severity of Sleep Disorders. Strengthening the orbicularis oris (lip and mouth) muscles will replace mouth breathing and prompt nose breathing.

I bought a Lip Trainer in 2015 and was glad I did. Given that it's a development that can catalyse profound changes in people, the Lip Trainer has been wholeheartedly embraced by doctors, dentists and hospitals throughout Asia.

Pressure Points of the Body

Acupressure can relieve toothache pain and plays a vital role in overall health. Through gentle pressure, acupressure stimulates the meridians or energy channels that lead to the teeth and gums.

In the same way that the interactive tooth charts reveal which meridian is linked to which tooth, a basic knowledge of acupressure points on the body can help stimulate reactions as well as help offset any pain felt.

Toothpicks

Ancient Buddhist scriptures tell a story of Buddha throwing a used toothpick onto the ground and a Bodhi tree sprung up. So we know that toothpicks have been in use since the introduction of Buddhism in Japan.

The use of toothpicks in Asia is commonplace, yet in the West, the habit seems to have been lost. One Western dentist suggested that toothpick use is a downright dangerous practice, but I would suggest that common sense contributes to their proper use....gently. If you impale your gum with a toothpick, you only have yourself to blame. Use wooden toothpicks, as plastic ones often end up floating in our oceans!

Temporo Mandibular Joint

The temporomandibular joint (TMJ) is the joint of the jaw that helps you move your lower jaw (mandible) up and down. Your mandible is the strongest bone in your head*.

* Despite the incorrect answer given in the board game Trivial Pursuit, the femur is the strongest bone in your body, not the mandible. The femur has a breaking strain of 400 kilos; the mandible has a breaking strain of 195 kilos. You should get extra Trivial Pursuit points for knowing this!

Only the lower jaw (mandible) moves during any motion, and your teeth will match correctly if the TMJ is stress-free. Prolonged anxiety compresses the TMJ, leading to muscle-contracting headaches.

The TMJ derived its name from the two bones that form the joint:

- the upper Temporal bone, which is part of the skull and
- the lower jaw bone, the Mandible (With thanks to F Gailliard for the TMJ image)

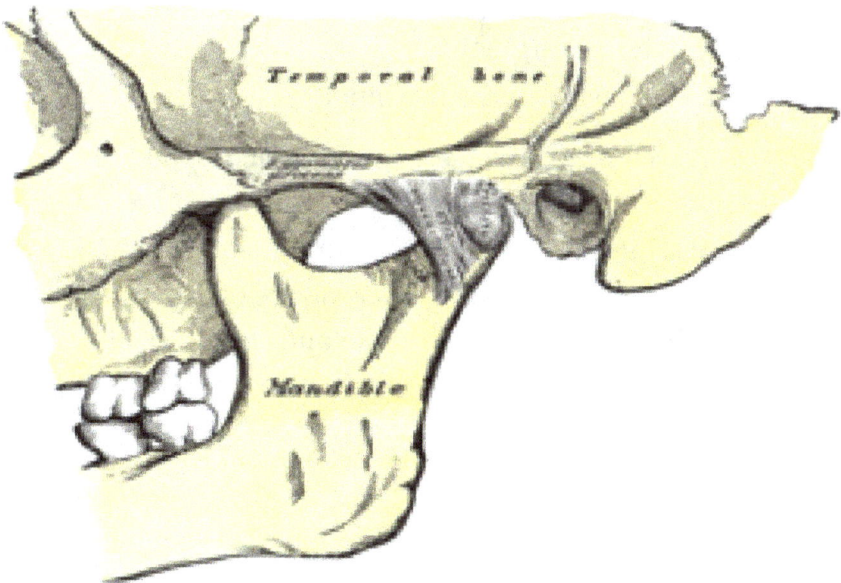

This crucial part of your body is affected by almost every other part of your body. All kinds of problems can result, such as headaches, toothaches, neck/shoulder pain, and even back pain or hamstring problems. Sadly, many dentists remain unaware of this whole-body connection as it wasn't part of their *'put me through the sausage machine'* training (as one newly qualified dentist described it to me).

Key into your browser: **Modern Reflexology: Acupressure Point For Jaw Pain And TMJ**

TMJ disorders are brought about by:

- Teeth grinding and teeth clenching
- Gum chewing or fingernail biting
- Misalignment of the teeth or fillings (malocclusion)
- Trauma (fractures) to the jaw or facial bones
- Occupational tasks eg. violinists, artists, hairdressers, switchboard operators
- Incorrect posture
- Orthodontic treatment
- Lack of breastfeeding as an infant

When you swallow, your teeth often touch. This sets off a neuromuscular trigger in your body. If your teeth are occluding incorrectly because a filling is too prominent, your body will quickly adjust itself, and you won't be aware of any adjustments. Over time, it will become chronic and may result in pain elsewhere in your body, but you will have no idea or memory of where it originated.

> *"The TMJ is the headquarters of the body's balance mechanism, and if the jaw doesn't close properly because of maloccluded teeth, the balance mechanism is forced to adapt. However, because it's under constant stress, the brain is*

pumping out lots of noradrenalin and serotonin. This sensitizes the autonomic nervous system, making the patient vulnerable to any other stressors like bad diet or emotional problems. So depression could be linked to TMJ dysfunction."

'What Doctors Don't Tell You' .

If your teeth are well-aligned, you can masticate and digest your food properly. It is, therefore, important that all restorations (fillings, inlays, crowns, bridgework....) are fitted with precision into these very delicate structures and do not cause any interference with other parts of your body.

One of the most effective treatments for supporting jawbone density and quality is CaviTau®. Hope your dentist has one.

Children's Teeth

A recent BBC report stated:

> *Dentists have accused the government of having a "short- sighted" approach to tooth decay in England after hospital operations to remove children's teeth increased to nearly 43,000. There were 42,911 operations in 2016-17 - up from 40,800 the previous year and 36,833 in 2012-13, NHS figures show.The British Dental Association said England had a "second-class" dental service compared to Wales and Scotland.*

> *The government said it was "determined" to reduce the number of extractions. Doctors said many of the tooth extractions would be caused by the food and drink children consume and were therefore"completely preventable".*

Dental surgeon Claire Stevens, who works in a hospital in north-west England, said most of her patients were aged five to nine, but it was not uncommon to remove all 20 baby teeth from a two-year-old because of decay.She said she has also extracted a 14-year-old's permanent teeth due to fizzy drinks. They then needed false teeth.

Whatever habits develop in childhood are often carried into adult years. I've always encouraged parents to start their children off with healthy brushing techniques. It's a way of saving children from developing poor brushing habits early on.

Accompanied by a song, children (and hopefully adults) will brush for longer than a minute, another good habit to develop. For the young ones - the Japanese Brush Your Teeth Song **Tokioheidi** is popular on YouTube. Follow along with the **Hamigaki song** (this is the Japanese version) at least you will have spent 2:44 mins brushing your teeth instead of the western average of 45 seconds!

Or there's the familiar **Sesame Street**. It's only a minute so play it twice.

Teenagers And Beyond

When your child becomes a teenager, musical choices go through a warp. I know. In my teen years, my parents generously put up with me listening to Frank Zappa/Mothers Of Invention, Jefferson Airplane, the Doors, Soft Machine, Cream and Pink Floyd - all without complaint!

Encourage your teenager to find a track for about 3 minutes. They'll willingly clean their teeth alone. Use YouTube to find these suggestions:

Green Day   **Pulling Teeth (2:31)**
Lorde   **White Teeth Teens (3:34)**
Megadeth   **Skin O' My Teeth (3:53)**

You may succeed more if you can encourage them to help you create a homemade mouthwash or toothpaste. Now, there's a real challenge.

Part Five:

Consider These Before Agreeing!

The purpose of what's written is to show you ways of keeping yourself free from unnecessary visits to the dentist's chair. Dentists are perfectly normal people with wives and children to feed, mortgages to pay and a ridiculous number of forms to fill out for government watchdogs. I have, therefore, put more effort into what's positive than what not to do. However, you'll have an uphill struggle if you don't know some of the pitfalls.

Oral Surgery

I list this first because it's becoming an increasingly common recommendation. To avoid gum surgery, necessary or otherwise, start making your own toothpaste and mouthwash at home. Use the ingredients you've just read about. Longer term, learn how to prevent gum disease and tooth decay from happening in the first place.....a much better option.

Surgery is carried out when people whose mouths have deteriorated to the extent that teeth may be falling out or their gums are in a dangerous condition. The majority of surgery is carried out for cosmetic reasons.

Despite this, Dr Joseph Phillips always warned his patients:

"No surgery has ever cured periodontal disease. Surgery shouldn't be done until the mouth is healthy; surgery being only a post healing reconstructive procedure."

Mercury & Amalgam

No prizes for guessing that a major cause of health problems in your body is induced by the mercury in your fillings. People suffering from mercury exposure may have Multiple Sclerosis, Alzheimer's and Parkinson's Diseases, Leukaemia, Arthritis, Diabetes, Seizures and the babies could suffer from birth defects. That's just a shortened list of the 200 mercury-related diseases documented by Dr. Hal Huggins. New evidence from the Dental Tribune suggests that mercury exposure from dental amalgams may also cause or contribute to depression, anxiety and suicide.

Author Bill Henderson believes there's a definite link between bungled dental work and cancer. He's known cancer patients to fully recover just by having their teeth fixed. He writes:

"While it's easy to figure out you need to have your mercury fillings and root-canaled teeth removed, it's not so easy to figure out who should do it. It's hard for a dentist to safely remove mercury fillings without releasing a large amount of mercury into the mouth and saliva. The patient runs the risk of inhaling mercury- contaminated vapor and swallowing mercury "down the hatch" into the stomach. There's a huge potential to take in more poison by having the fillings removed than by leaving them in place".

I had my mercury fillings removed by Dr Elmar Jung. To minimise any mercury vapour inhalation I was given an oxygen mask while Dr. Jung and the nurse wore Mercury Filter Masks.

In addition to this precaution Dr. Jung:

- ran a pre- and post-supplement regime, using specific suction procedures that shielded my body from ingesting any mercury particles or vapour,
- used an extra suction machine for any vapour released by drilling out the mercury fillings (my fillings weren't drilled out but instead broken into big chunks to reduce the chance of vapour exposure)
- gave me a high dose of Vitamin C i.v. infusion, and
- kept the practice windows wide open

Dr Jung also explained to me the steps to take in the weeks and months following the mercury removal. As mercury is a biochemical disaster within, have the mercury fillings removed from your mouth as a priority (especially children and pregnant women).

It is crucial to have mercury removed from both parents before conception, as the majority of holistic dentists would prefer not to perform this during pregnancy. Use the precautions Dr Jung took with me as a checklist for your dentist. The International Academy of Oral Medicine and Toxicology (IAOMT) Protocol is called S.M.A.R.T.

Amalgam used by dentists is a mix of metals consisting of liquid mercury and a powdered alloy from copper, silver and tin.

Up to 50% of dental amalgam is elemental mercury, one of many heavy metals we are exposed to daily!

These metals interfere with our proteins and enzymes, which in turn damage neurological functions (confusion, fatigue, memory loss), the kidneys, and the liver, all of which are crucial for the body to function as it should.

Dr. Tim O'Shea (The Doctor Within) writes:

"Today it's become more and more commonplace for people to be looking for a dentist who will remove mercury fillings. Many of the more conscientious dentists no longer use these amalgams, opting instead for the safer, more biocompatible ceramics and composites."

It is still illegal for a US dentist to suggest amalgam removal to a patient. This is dental politics. Such a suggestion might call into question the safety and therapeutic ethics of ADA's century-long policy of permanently installing the third most toxic substance known to man into the human oral cavity.

However, any dentist may remove the amalgams if the patient requests it. As the connection between mercury and many epidemic diseases becomes better known, the market for amalgam removal has taken a sharp upturn in recent years.

It doesn't matter what anyone in the Government tells you; no amount of mercury is safe within a human or animal body. Even the WHO concurs.

How is it possible for any health authority to admit that mercury is a poison and at the same time tell you it is 'harmless'?

In fairness to your well-meaning dentist, there's a pernicious control that runs through the industry.

"Unfortunately, conventional dentistry has something called the 'gag rule' – that means dentists

can't talk about the safety of dental amalgams in the dental chair without expecting criticism or worse from the dental boards."

Dr David Kennedy, DDS, Past President of the International Academy of Oral Medicine and Toxicology

We might ask why the US Multiple Sclerosis Society has remained staunchly averse to even considering mercury as a cause of the debilitating condition, at one point actively campaigning against investigating the mercury issue. It's based on that old chestnut, 'follow the money.'

Chuck Rekoske, former Chairman of the Kansas MS Society and an MS sufferer, decided to have his amalgam fillings removed. He improved to the extent that he could play 3 sets of tennis each day with his son. When Chuck started recommending amalgam removal the society invited him to resign for "conflict of interest". Enough said there!

- - - - -

STOP PRESS - email received on 30 May 2024 from Charlie Brown, President, World Alliance for Mercury-Free Dentistry.

As the European Council explains in its recent press release:

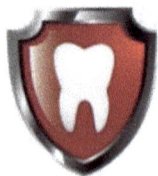

"Today, the Council adopted a regulation to completely ban the use of dental amalgams... The regulation will now be signed and published in the Official Journal of the EU. It will enter into force on the twentieth day following publication and become directly applicable in all member states."

You may be aware that the European Council and Parliament struck a deal to end the amalgam era in February 2023. Now this deal has been formally adopted as the law of the land!

With this new regulation, we win four major victories...

- Amalgam use ends in all EU countries on 1 January 2025 (with only narrow exemptions that will be up for review by the end of 2029).
- Amalgam manufacture in the EU is phased out as of 1 July 2026.
- Amalgam exports from the EU are banned as of 1 January 2025.
- Amalgam imports into the EU are banned as of 1 July 2026.

It took more than a decade of our intense campaigning – from countless hearings and meetings with government officials to reams of comments and scientific evidence.

We could not have done it without the energy of our many supporters.

Thanks to you, this toxic mercury product is now officially banned in all 27 EU countries!

Stay tuned as we push governments in the United States, Canada, Australia, New Zealand and UK to follow suit!

Charles G Brown

Fluoride

Sources of Fluoride

- Toothpaste enhanced with fluoride
- Fluoridated Water Supplies
- Mouthwash enhanced with fluoride
- Food processed with fluoridated water
- Fluoride Supplements

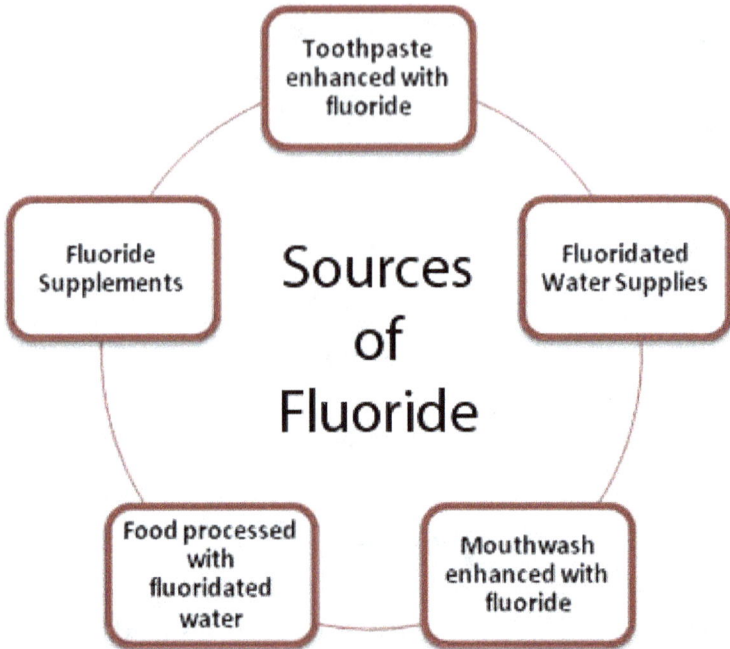

Fluoridated water is unquestionably a massive mandatory medication, using the endorsement of government health departments and dentists to propagate the myth that it helps to prevent tooth decay; public water supplies/reservoirs and bottled water are the drug delivery systems of choice. Why do they bother to claim that fluoride is there to protect your teeth when 70% of tooth loss is caused by gum disease? This rationale doesn't even pass the laugh test.

In his award-winning documentary Fluoridegate: An American Tragedy, Dr. David Kennedy sounded the alarm against fluoridation. According to the official description:

> *"This film reveals how government, industry and trade associations protect and promote a policy*

known to cause harm to our country and especially to small children who suffer more than any other segment of the population. While their motivation remains uncertain, the outcome is crystal clear: it is destroying our nation!"

In his report *"Why Fluoride Is Toxic"*, renowned doctor and neurosurgeon Dr. Russell Blaylock explains how we are all being lied to about the safety of artificial fluoride in our water. Repeated claims by government health authorities that fluoride is completely safe ignore copious scientific evidence pointing to both brain and nervous system damage in conjunction with fluoride exposure, not to mention an elevated risk of cancer.

Of the many threats to the health of your mouth, brain, thyroid, nervous system, kidneys, and pineal gland, fluoride is one of the greatest.

A groundbreaking new study in Mexico found that exposure to fluoride during pregnancy can harm IQ and cognitive development in children. The kids are our future. Stop dumbing them down!

How To Minimise Fluoride Exposure

A quality water filter installed in your home can help eliminate, or at least reduce, the amount of fluoride you and your family are exposed to daily. Stop using fluoride toothpaste. Supplement instead with iodine as it helps the body to purge accumulations of fluoride, chlorine and bromine as well as heavy metals (aluminium, mercury, lead and cadmium). 96% of Americans are iodine deficient.

World's Oldest and Best Known Peer Reviewed Medical Journal

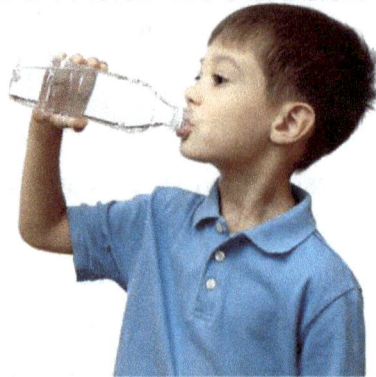

Officially Classifies Fluoride
as a Neurotoxin.

Chances are you are too. Iodine in your body is vital to your overall health. Be very wary about eating seafood caught in the Pacific. The damaging effects from Fukushima have not been remedied - they've only been suppressed.

There are a range of good water filters that facilitate the removal of fluoride, chlorine, and other additives from water. As it could be one of the best investments you'll ever make, I recommend searching for what's affordable in your country.

Nerve Extractions

In his book "Covering the Nerve Removal," Dr George Meinig wrote:

> *"... when infected teeth produce disorders in other parts of the body, the infection does not necessarily*

have to be great, but the evidence suggests that dangerous poisons can come from infected teeth to the lymphatic system or blood, or both, producing a disorder much worse than infection. Evidence suggests that poisonous substances can, under certain conditions, reduce the sensitivity of the organism or special tissues, so that smaller amounts of toxin-producing organisms can produce a larger reaction and disorder. "

This may underscore why a nerve removal operation is not to be considered lightly. Whenever a nerve is extracted from a tooth, the bacteria within that tooth continue to produce harmful toxins that can cause poor health conditions. Systemic damage may occur if these infections and toxins are not detected in time.

As the removal of a nerve effectively kills the tooth, the human body rejects it as it instinctively rejects other dead tissue. The tooth without a nerve will become the underlying cause of any subsequent infections.

Think of it as a gangrene. A 'carrier' may suffer for many years without knowing they are carrying what is termed 'focal' infections. Infected bacteria or their toxins from this area may migrate throughout the entire body, in turn transferring the toxins to other organs or contributing to heart attacks, strokes, liver and kidney damage.

Although the complete removal of the tooth may unbalance the jaw, this option may be the better alternative. Discuss this with your dentist.

X-Rays

Not all dental problems are obvious or create recognisable symptoms, so let's side with the dentist. X-rays have tremendous value in the early detection of dental disease and can make a huge difference in the treatment recommended. Without the aid of an X-ray, your dentist's ability to diagnose is restricted.

If your dentist needs to take an X-ray, make 100% sure a lead-lined thyroid or bodyguard is used to protect you from radiation during the procedure. Thankfully, with modern X-rays, the radiation needed to create images goes directly to where it's aimed.

Just before an x-ray some years ago, I asked my (then) dentist for a thyroid guard. He admitted that his practice had recently been bought by a group of accountants, and the lead guards had all been sold as no one asked for them!

Unfortunately, GDC guidelines say people don't need any lead protection during X-rays. What qualifications in stupidity were they awarded?

If you ask your dentist about the safety of X-ray equipment, the reply you'll get will be "quite safe." They'll probably change the subject by comparing it with the safety of air travel, but with an X-ray, you get the radiation exposure in one hit rather than over the duration of the flight.

You know, and I know that this comparison is nonsense, so look your dentist in the eye and say you saw exactly the same model of the x-ray machine about to be used on display in the Victoria and Albert Museum last year. The reply you get next may be a little more honest.

If you want to sound less of an easy target, be very clear about the radiation levels an X-ray will expose you to. Tell your dentist that recent findings from an Oxford University study demonstrate that even lower doses of radiation than those used in X-rays and CT scans can cause cancer. Your dentist's reply will be interesting. If you add, "I'm aware of the cumulative effect of repeated exposure to ionizing radiation", you may be treated with more respect.

Avoid unnecessary X-rays wherever possible.

Root Canal Treatments

Here's a treatment your dentist will likely recommend, telling you is perfectly safe. But there may be a banana skin in this procedure waiting for you to step on.

The reality is that people want to save their teeth even after infection sets in. Root canals are the standard 'next step' even though extracting teeth can cause other problems, such as a shift in a person's bite as well as other unwanted health issues.

So what's the answer?

One of the goals is to re-establish the periodontal ligament surrounding the root of the tooth. This is a membrane around the root that acts like a shock absorber that has secondary blood supply and nerve supply. Yet once a tooth has been root-treated it is dead and should be removed.

In my opinion there is no such thing as a 'healthy' root canal treatment.

If it were me, my preference would be to have a bridge or an implant with a non-metallic substance such as Zirconia. More expensive, but the alternative is not worth considering.

The challenge is keeping the tooth free of bacteria, which is nigh impossible. The moment you stop using any prevention agents or frequencies, bacteria will simply migrate back into the tooth, hiding somewhere in the 4 - 6 miles of tubular channels therein, excreting their toxins into your body.

The movie **"Root Cause"** was shown on Netflix but in 2019 pressure forced Netflix to remove it from their library without any explanation given.

Dr George Meinig wrote extensively on the hazards of root canal work:

If your dentist ever recommends a root canal, key into your browser: **The 3 1/2 Year Success of 'Root Canal Cover-Up' By George E. Meinig**

The story in the link below is worth listening to. You may see a red warning page designed to scare you into not opening the link. This is just a form of censorship. If you're hesitant just make sure not to download anything. I've opened it many times.

Find this video on YouTube: **Before It's News: You Won't Believe How Root Canals Affect Your Entire Body (1:15:37)**

We mustn't lose sight of the experiments Dr Weston Price carried out in the early 1900's when he became suspicious that root canal teeth were creating degenerative diseases in his patients.

Whether he implanted the entire tooth or a portion of the tooth under the skin of a laboratory animal, the animal, usually a rabbit, would almost always develop the same disease as the patient. Most of the rabbits died within two weeks because the infections proved so devastating.

Root canal treatments are at best a 'quick fix' option if you are in excruciating pain. There can be consequences, but it may not be for years after the event that you start to suffer from them. Any link between the root canal and the consequent result will be emphatically denied.

The American Dental Association claims root canals have been proven safe. The trouble is they have NO reliable research to substantiate this claim. Read on if you've had root canal work or have been recommended such treatment.

Hal Huggins was the dentist who was the most responsible for educating the the public about mercury's toxicity in dental amalgams. He wrote:

> *"Bacteria will always find a way to continue to infect the tooth and if you get a root canal procedure your mouth could become a safe haven for some really nasty bad guys. So instead of drilling and sealing, pulling the tooth and replacing it with a fake tooth - eventual bonded and bridged - is the way to go."*

Natural Society writes:

> *"A root canal essentially removes the live pulp from a tooth and replaces it with a synthetic material. This stops the tooth from appearing to rot away, it does rot away with the internal damage that could be causing a toothache, the damage from an untreated cavity. But, while your*

dentist would have you think the root canal solves your problems - it really isn't that simple.

In addition to the central root of the tooth, where the dentist removes the tissue during a root canal, there are thousands of tiny side canals that aren't removed touched. They rot. They fester and become a breeding ground for bacteria and infection. Research has proven this to be the case."

The amount of these tiny side canals left untouched can add up to 2-3 miles per tooth. When a root canal is performed, the dentist hollows out the tooth before filling out the hollow chamber with a substance that cuts off the tooth from its blood supply. At that point, fluid can no longer circulate through the tooth. Yet the honeycomb maze of tubules remains. When bacteria that do not require oxygen (anaerobic) are cut off from their food supply, they hide in these tunnels where they're safe from antibiotics and your immune defences.

"The toxins created by root canals are more toxic than botulism"
Dr. Thomas Levy

After a root canal is performed, the tooth is dead. Whenever a body organ dies, it is always removed before it can do any damage. Why on earth would anyone want a dead tooth left in their mouth for the rest of their life? Especially as a root-canal-treated tooth inevitably becomes infected, often chronically.

Why does this not become painful? Because the nerve complex has been surgically removed, such pain can no longer be felt - even when the tooth is mutely screaming at the rest of the body about the potent pathogens multiplying therein.

Unfortunately, a dead tooth will continue to discharge toxins into your body with no discernible symptoms - no pain, no swellings - nothing to alert you that it is wreaking havoc upon your immune system, causing chronic and acute medical conditions. Being surgically blocked off from entering the mouth, these toxins are released into the lymphatic system and enter venous blood from the jawbones, where they accumulate before spreading throughout the body.

A 26-person case study published in the American Academy of Periodontology (1998) concluded that all subjects' root canal sites and blood samples contained anaerobic bacteria. It's a safe bet that a never-ending stream of bacteria starts flowing into your bloodstream from the minute you are given that root canal.

Cancer specialist Dr. Josef Issels, MD (1907 – 1998), asked all of his cancer patients to have their dead teeth removed. In his book 'Cancer: A Second Opinion', he explains that he has worked with 16,000 cancer patients over 40 years, and some 90% of his patients had a dead tooth or teeth in their mouths. The link between the mouth and cancer was clear. In addition to that, a Swiss Cancer Clinic found that of 150 patients suffering from breast cancer, 147 of them had one or more root canal-treated teeth, some of them on the same acupuncture meridian as the cancerous breast.

What are your choices?

Discuss having the tooth pulled with your dentist. Yes, this might compromise the balance of the jaw, but it's still likely to be a better option than the root canal. An alternative approach of using stem cells to regrow your teeth is being researched.

Although this is still a specialty area and unlikely to be available from high-street dentists for a while, this is a discussion you need to have with your dentist.

Wisdom Tooth Removal

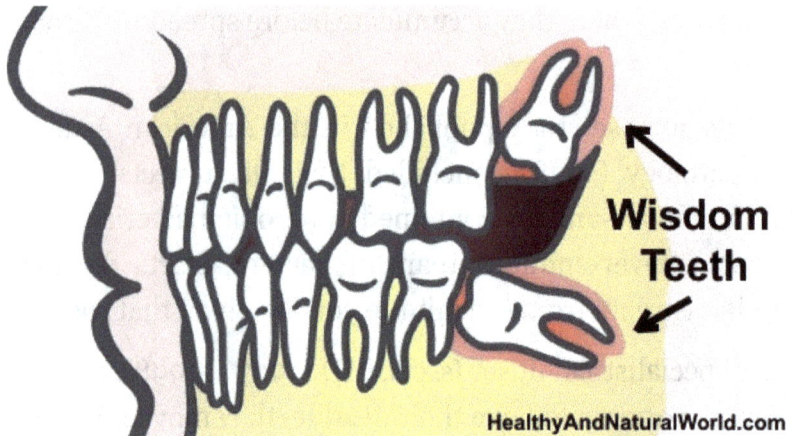

HealthyAndNaturalWorld.com

If you're told your child should have four healthy teeth removed to create more space, know that THIS IS NONSENSE. Firstly, no more space is created and the treatment with fixed braces can be massively traumatic.

Wisdom Teeth or Third Molars, are the teeth at the back of your mouth. They usually develop or 'erupt' in your late teens or early twenties.

It turns out that there's growing evidence that the removal procedure is rarely justified.

67% of all wisdom teeth extractions are medically unnecessary. Tooth extraction disrupts the flow of neuro-transmitters and breaks the acupuncture meridians, which have a vital relationship between our teeth and our entire body including bones, joints, organs and endocrine glands.

I still have my wisdom teeth. Whew!

In the early days of dentistry wisdom teeth were only removed in times of real trouble. Back then, people were eating better quality food, and wisdom teeth erupted properly into their mouths. Nowadays, with fast foods and sugary drinks, jaws aren't developing as they should (remember Dr Weston Price and his findings with Indigenous tribes?).

After the Second World War, the number of practicing dentists increased, and the recommendation to remove wisdom teeth suddenly became a 'precautionary measure'.

There are of course genuine reasons for removing wisdom teeth, such as when a tooth has become ingrown, impacted or decayed. Failure to remove the tooth in these cases can lead to infections and considerable pain, although that isn't always the case for 3 million+ people every year in the USA who have their wisdom teeth extracted at the recommendation of their dentist.

Extracting wisdom teeth can be very painful and upset the balance of the jaw as well as causing cheek numbness and even broken jaws. People are known to have gone into a coma or, sadly, died during the procedure. Serious consequences, in particular, are true in adolescence when the wisdom tooth roots are still forming. So the possibility exists that more complications can result from the surgery than from leaving the wisdom teeth where they are.

If you are faced with a wisdom tooth removal choice, I suggest you speak with a good cranio-sacral therapist. Cranial work can help relieve restrictions within the jaw and restore mobility without resorting to surgery.

You'll be told that the teeth have not fully 'erupted' into position and are still covered by gum tissue or jawbone and that complications may follow if nothing is done immediately. Some dentists even claim that wisdom teeth are simply unnecessary teeth that crowd out your mouth. Now you know better!

Retired dentist Dr. Jay Friedman, DDS, dispelled the myths surrounding wisdom teeth extractions, suggesting that two-thirds of them are not necessary and should be classified as a public health hazard.

DO NOT BE PRESSURED into having your wisdom teeth removed. Know that most wisdom teeth can be left the way they are.

If we revisit Dr. Weston Price's work for a moment, he concluded that proper nutrition is the basis of dental and overall health. Holistic dentists understand the simple fact that when you supply sufficient nutrients to the jaw bone during its development, all 32 teeth will have sufficient space to develop without any over-crowding. Of course, it does help if both your parents have a good set of teeth.

Inappropriate recommendations from your dentist are as welcome as a porcupine at a nudist colony. I'm quoting an extract from Health Ranger Mike Adams's newsletter, as many of us will face the same problem.

He writes:

> *"I don't trust dentists. I've long suspected dentists of scaring patients into undergoing unnecessary procedures in order to generate more business. My suspicions were confirmed when I visited a dentist in 2001 for a basic checkup. After taking dental x-rays (another health hazard, as new research is showing), my dentist fed me a scare story about*

how I still had all my wisdom teeth, and that all those teeth needed to be surgically removed. I was absolutely stunned.

My wisdom teeth were working just fine: no cavities, no pain, no problems. I had made an appointment for a routine checkup, not to undergo expensive surgery for my wisdom teeth. But my dentist insisted, relying on a variety of scare tactics to try to convince me to undergo this expensive -- and completely unnecessary procedure. His behavior was highly unethical. He was using his authority and position as "the dentist" to try to scare me into accepting a surgical procedure that I quite obviously didn't need.

In fact, even he couldn't give me a good reason for justifying the surgery other than to say, "We usually remove the wisdom teeth quite early." Which means, of course, that they just order the surgery for every child or teenager who walks into the clinic, regardless of whether they actually need it.

Now, it turns out, the removal of wisdom teeth has been found to be an utterly worthless procedure to begin with. It *"may do more harm than good"* says the British Medical Journal, after reviewing literally thousands of case studies.

So the dentist is really just hyping an unnecessary procedure, and if your dentist is anything like some dentists I've encountered, they're also using all sorts of highly unethical scare tactics to try to force people into undergoing the procedure. That's downright bad for the profession, yet it's a common practice among dentists in the United States."

RFID chips

Scientists in Belgium have successfully embedded an RFID chip into a tooth to store personal information. Their reasoning is that it allows forensic teams to identify a person in the event of a natural disaster. Nice try, guys, but the real reason is about controlling the masses. They want to know where you are every minute of the day and night.

I saw "The Matrix" too. I would consider this action to be no less than an un-consented assault.

Whatever the truth is about embedding RFID chips in teeth, the insertion of microchips into human beings (aka Revelations 'Mark Of The Beast') is gaining momentum in the USA, Canada, and Europe. To distract us, we're shown videos on how easy, painless, and useful these microchip implants will be in making us safer....and opening office doors easier!

Given that microchips in pets are already a known cause of cancer, we all have to be on alert so RFID chips are not inserted into us unwillingly.

Sports Drinks: Nothing 'sporty' about them

Those of you who keep fit need to know that heavy exercising has a downside:

1. **Sports drinks** are heavily promoted to convince exercise enthusiasts they're a healthy way to replace electrolytes lost during training. Marketing sleight of mouth there. Sports drinks don't quench your thirst; they actually slow down hydration. In addition

- you're probably swallowing more calories (sugar) than you just burned off
- the high sugar content cancels out any electrolyte benefits
- there's zero protein in sports drinks. Bad news for muscle builders.
- high sugar levels usually cause a subsequent energy crash

The Academy of General Dentistry published the results of a study which measured the high acid content in sports drinks. The report evidenced that damage occurs to the body after only 5 days of consistent consumption. The lead author of the study, Poonam Jain, BDS, MS, MPH, wrote:

> *"Young adults consume these drinks assuming that they will improve their sports performance and energy levels and that they are 'better' for them than soda. Most of these patients are shocked to learn that these drinks are essentially bathing their teeth with acid."*

Another study at the dental school of University Hospital Heidelberg, Germany, concluded that athletes tended to have more cavities as training time increased. The more hours an athlete spent exercising and training, the more likely they were to develop a cavity. The reason? It's linked with what comes next....

2. **Nose Breathing:** I mentioned earlier the benefits of nose breathing over mouth breathing. While exercising, people tend to breathe through an open mouth. The result is the mouth drying out, a reduced saliva flow and a more favourable environment in which bacteria can flourish. Nose breathing on the other hand produces nitric oxide

which crucially increases the ability of your lungs to absorb oxygen. The bonus is that, at the same time, it lowers your blood pressure.

If you want to get more benefits from exercising, drink pure water or coconut water. If you want your water to be flavoured, add a slice of lemon or a pinch of unrefined sea salt, but don't go fizzy!

Another case for using the Lip Trainer.

What Else Are You Drinking?

It's those fizzy drinks that knock you back. No question. I know they're more-ish but would you drink a can with the word POISON written on it? OK, 'POISON' harms you quickly, and these drinks cause their damage slowly, so there is a difference. The consistent word here is 'harm'. So I'll rephrase that to "Would you drink a can that had the words 'The Contents Of This Drink Will Harm You Slowly" on the bottle?"

Your parents told you about fizzy drinks, and I've just reminded you. It's up to you from now on! Two ingredients, citric acid and phosphoric acid, provide the tangy sensation. They make it taste refreshing, but as they pass through your mouth, they slowly damage your enamel, the protector of your teeth.

I'm not being puritan here. OK, maybe a little, as I drank Coke as a kid. The last can of Coke (or was it Pepsi?) I drank was, I believe, in about 1995. An occasional fizzy drink won't tip the scales, but if you're in the habit of drinking them regularly, you'll become one of your dentist's most valued patients.

The enamel on your teeth will soften, and you'll become more susceptible to tooth decay and gum disease. This won't pose an immediate concern when you're young, but when the dental bills add up in middle age, you'll wish things had gone differently.

Drink more water. Drink green and black tea to reduce plaque build-up and help balance bacteria levels in the mouth.

As sugar fuels acidity and creates an uneven ratio of bacteria in your mouth, manage your intake sensibly. It's often said that if sugar were invented today, it would be banned, but the Church and State have made so much money from it that it's actively promoted! Look how many shops have sweets and chocolates on display at their checkout counters for impulse buyers, especially if you're queueing with children.

Sugar is what accelerates the formation of plaque. It's this plaque that eats away at your enamel. Not just that - studies in Copenhagen in 2016 evidenced that in addition to reducing sperm count, consuming colas could impact erectile function.

If you have children, get them to sip carbonated drinks through a straw to keep the acid away from their teeth. Even with sparkling water.

Smoking

This is not a tirade to tell you about the hazards of smoking. That was your parents' job. Given what we know about the short, medium and long-term effects of smoking, I'm surprised that anyone does it today. But that's just me.

I raise the issue only as a reminder that smoking contributes to tooth staining, gum disease, and tooth loss and can, in severe cases, cause oral cancers. I imagine this isn't news to you.

What you may not be aware of is that smoking can also increase bone loss within the jaw, impair the benefits of dental surgery, slow down recovery processes within the mouth and inflame the salivary glands. Just saying!

Chewing Gum

In the mid-1970s, I travelled up the Belait River in Brunei, Borneo, with friends. I have an enduring memory of a small wooden construction elevated above the river bank at the confluence with the Mendaram River. In the building, several elderly women were chewing away on something. Here were the "chewing gum ladies," using their mouths to soften the gum base before it was processed into chewing gum.

I haven't unwrapped a stick of chewing gum for several decades, yet every time I see someone chewing gum, it triggers this indelible memory of its potential origins.

Historically the gum base was sourced from natural tree resins, the flavours extracted from natural herbs and spices. Today, it's a different story as many popular chewing gum brands are loaded with plastics, rubbers and synthetic or GMO sweetening components.

Millions of people use gum daily to freshen their breath. But many chewing gums are so packed with toxins that, if you knew what was in them, you'd think seriously before unwrapping another strip. Repeated gum chewing weakens the digestive aspects of your saliva. So, if you eat a meal after chewing gum for a couple of hours, the digestive strength of your saliva will be lost.

Chewing sends a signal that food is coming. If digestive enzymes are insufficient to break down the food, gut tissue is required to carry out this function. This can damage the gut if repeated over a long period.

Chewing gum may be among the toxic foods we can legally buy. Common carcinogenic ingredients include Butylated Hydroxytoluene, Titanium Dioxide, plasticisers, fillers, resins, and elastomers.

Add to that Aspartame (linked to brain tumours, cancers, diabetes, neurological disorders and birth defects; acesulfame potassium (similar to aspartame), sorbitol/xylitol/mannitol (sugar alcohols altered enough to be considered "sugar-free legally.").

If there aren't enough cancer-causing ingredients listed above to put you off gum, the chewing motion itself can cause long-term wear and tear to the jawbone cartilage. Its purpose is to be a shock absorber, so you need to keep it in working order, especially when you're older. Lose that protective feature, and jaw movements become painful.

I've been repeatedly told that "the best way" to reduce the rogue bacteria in your mouth is to use (sugar substitute) Xylitol chewing gum or Xylitol toothpaste. This may surprise some of you, as Xylitol had a good name for years. Those halcyon years were probably when Xylitol was extracted from birch bark; today it's GMO corn.

Xylitol is an anti-cariogenic (foods with constituent parts that carry beneficial effects that inhibit the development of cavities), but it can be toxic. Animal testing has evidenced that Xylitol can be lethal to animals, so be careful what you put in your and your children's mouths.

Either buy natural gum or snack on organic liquorice sticks instead. They're bacteria-killing and prevent oral infections.

If you have amalgam fillings, chewing gum releases between 4 and 40 micrograms of mercury each day. Drinking hot drinks, eating food, and even brushing your teeth contribute to this vapour release as well.

Baby's Milk Bottles

Watching a baby suckle on its mother's breast, it's easy to get the impression that the baby is exerting gentle pressure on its mother's nipple. The first milk bottles for babies were constructed with this belief.

This failed to recreate a baby's natural suction, presuming that they massage the milk using a peristaltic wave motion, pressing the nipple up against the roof of the mouth. Recent ultrasound images convey that the baby is, in fact, creating a vacuum to extract milk.

Be careful when you buy food containers or baby milk bottles. The synthetic chemical Bisphenol A (aka BPA) is a potent, oestrogen-mimicking compound used in everything from dental sealants for children's teeth to the linings of metal food cans and the thermal paper used for cash register receipts.

Frederick vom Saal, Professor of Biology at the University of Missouri, has become the harshest critic of corporate USA and the health regulators for actively concealing the dangers that exposure to BPA is clearly having on human health - from an increased risk of prostate cancer to heart disease and damage to the reproductive system. BPA was removed from all products in Japan ten years ago.

BPA contains gender-bending chemicals and is used in many plastics as well as being sprayed on foods (in the form of

Atrazine). It's a chemical castration. Ever wondered what's causing the explosion of transgenderism?

Make sure you only buy certified BPA-free bottles.

Baby teeth

In 2015, 33,000 children were admitted to a UK hospital with rotting teeth and, in many cases, had teeth removed under general anaesthetic. Deterioration is likely to have started when the children were infants.

The best thing you can do for your baby is to stay away from high-sugar fruit juices (READ THOSE LABELS) and ensure plaque has no time to become activated after meals, especially after carbohydrates (starches and sugars) meals. Teething rusks are great for babies, especially when teething, but they leave a residue which coats the emerging teeth.

> *"I think brushing is important, but not activating plaque with simple sugars is more important,"* Dr. Kevin Boyd

The argument over when to introduce solids has been going on for years, with highly qualified physicians and research scientists differing. The answer may be quite straightforward. It takes approximately 18 months for a baby's digestive system to develop. 9 months in utero and 9 months as a newborn.

If you introduce solids before the digestive tract is ready, willing and able, there's a significant risk of the baby developing an early allergy to those first foods. That's not rocket science.

Amongst the most common adult allergies is NUTS - especially peanuts. When breastfeeding, some mothers develop nipple rash.

To offset the inflammation and skin cracking, a nipple cream is applied before feeding. What is the base oil in many of those creams? Peanut oil. They've spent millions researching this particular allergy in adults. You got that from me for free!

Where I've mentioned articles, videos or even products, below you'll find links that help you understand or access these recommendations.

Graeme Dinnen

Graeme Dinnen
ResourcesForLife.net

Recommended Reading

'Shut Your Mouth And Open Wide'
Dr Elmar Jung

In a refreshingly entertaining, jaw-dropping, sometimes shocking way, Dr Jung drills into the root causes of dental health issues. You'll learn about hazardous toxins, life-threatening risks of dental materials and dental some questionable treatments ....and what you can do about them. An extremely readable and popular book you can order from most book websites.

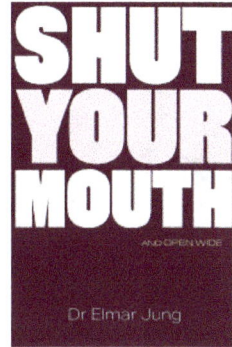

Recommended Products

Celtic Sea Salt	UK	ResourcesForLife.net
(Unrefined)	USA/Canada	SelinaNaturally.com
	Australia	saltoftheearth.com.au

Use YouTube to watch this clip

Your Teeth, Your Health: A New Perspective with Dorte Bredgaard (32.25)

The video from Danish Dentist Dirty Bredgaard gives us a fresh if somewhat unusual perspective. As I listened to her speak I realised what value she has to contribute to what we might classify as 'alternative' dentistry. This should be considered by anyone training in dental school. Diseases are 'the language of the teeth'. When we understand what the teeth are saying, then it's possible to spot and transform unsuitable patterns and make enriching life changes that can be felt in your everyday life (as well as in your bank account).

Things To Remember

1. Drink clean water to flush bacteria off your teeth. This reduces the risk of gum disease, and helps with fewer cavities and fresher breath. I swish water around my mouth as if I was 'oil pulling'.
2. Work these into your weekly routine: Iodine - Unrefined Celtic Sea Salt - Activated Charcoal - Bicarbonate of Soda - Coconut Oil
3. Reduce or eliminate flossing. Only use floss (very gently) to remove food that's trapped between your teeth. Even then be extremely careful not to cut your gum.
4. 7-Day Challenge: You have seven days starting today to make your first batch of homemade toothpaste and mouthwash. On your marks, get set...

Congratulations on reaching the end. Our thanks for buying this book. If you benefitted in any way, please feel free to leave an informative review. Your contribution will help others with challenges to their oral health.

If you don't have time to write anything, simply login to your Amazon page and press the star rating offered there.

Main amazon.com page
www.amazon.com/dp/B0CW1GD4CJ

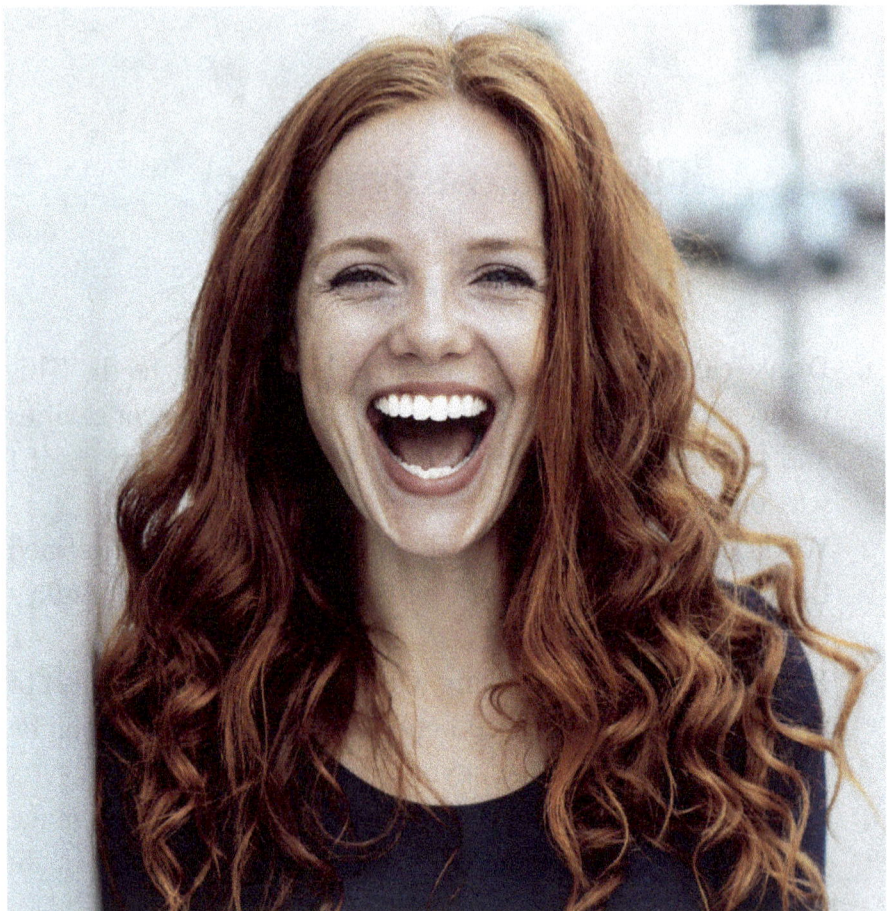

Be proud of your smile.....